T0259505

Otology and Otic Disease

Editors

BRADLEY L. NJAA
LYNETTE K. COLE

VETERINARY CLINICS OF NORTH AMERICA: SMALL ANIMAL PRACTICE

www.vetsmall.theclinics.com

November 2012 • Volume 42 • Number 6

ELSEVIER

1600 John F. Kennedy Blvd. • Suite 1800 • Philadelphia, PA 19103-2899
http://www.vetsmall.theclinics.com

**VETERINARY CLINICS OF NORTH AMERICA: SMALL ANIMAL PRACTICE Volume 42, Number 6
November 2012 ISSN 0195-5616, ISBN-13: 978-1-4557-4971-3**

Editor: John Vassallo; j.vassallo@elsevier.com

Veterinary Clinics of North America: Small Animal Practice (ISSN 0195-5616) is published bimonthly (For Post Office use only: volume 42 issue 1 of 6) by Elsevier Inc., 360 Park Avenue South, New York, NY 10010-1710. Months of issue are January, March, May, July, September, and November. Business and Editorial Offices: 1600 John F. Kennedy Blvd., Ste. 1800, Philadelphia, PA 19103-2899. Customer Service Office: 3251 Riverport Lane, Maryland Heights, MO 63043. Periodicals postage paid at New York, NY and additional mailing offices. Subscription prices are $283.00 per year (domestic individuals), $455.00 per year (domestic institutions), $138.00 per year (domestic students/residents), $375.00 per year (Canadian individuals), $559.00 per year (Canadian institutions), $416.00 per year (international individuals), $559.00 per year (international institutions), and $201.00 per year (international and Canadian students/residents). To receive student/resident rate, orders must be accompanied by name of affiliated institution, date of term, and the *signature* of program/residency coordinator on institution letterhead. Orders will be billed at individual rate until proof of status is received. Foreign air speed delivery is included in all *Clinics* subscription prices. All prices are subject to change without notice. **POSTMASTER:** Send address changes to *Veterinary Clinics of North America: Small Animal Practice*, Elsevier Health Sciences Division, Subscription Customer Service, 3251 Riverport Lane, Maryland Heights, MO 63043. Customer Service (orders, claims, online, change of address): Elsevier Periodicals Customer Service, Elsevier Health Sciences Division Subscription Customer Service 3251 Riverport Lane Maryland Heights, MO 63043. Tel: 1-800-654-2452 (U.S. and Canada); 314-447-8871 (outside U.S. and Canada). Fax: 314-447-8029. E-mail: journalscustomerservice-usa@elsevier.com (for print support); journalsonlinesupport-usa@elsevier.com (for online support). *Reprints.* For copies of 100 or more of articles in this publication, please contact the Commercial Reprints Department, Elsevier Inc., 360 Park Avenue South, New York, NY 10010-1710. Tel.: 212-633-3812; Fax: 212-462-1935; E-mail: reprints@elsevier.com.

Veterinary Clinics of North America: Small Animal Practice is also published in Japanese by Inter Zoo Publishing Co., Ltd., Aoyama Crystal-Bldg 5F, 3-5-12 Kitaaoyama, Minato-ku, Tokyo 107-0061, Japan.

Veterinary Clinics of North America: Small Animal Practice is covered in *Current Contents/Agriculture, Biology and Environmental Sciences, Science Citation Index, ASCA, MEDLINE/PubMed (Index Medicus), Excerpta Medica, and BIOSIS.*

Printed and bound by CPI Group (UK) Ltd, Croydon, CR0 4YY

Transferred to digital print 2012

Contributors

GUEST EDITORS

BRADLEY L. NJAA, DVM, MVSc
Diplomate, American College of Veterinary Pathologists; Associate Professor of Veterinary Pathology, Department of Veterinary Pathobiology, Center for Veterinary Health Sciences, Oklahoma State University, Stillwater, Oklahoma

LYNETTE K. COLE, DVM, MS
Diplomate, American College of Veterinary Dermatology; Associate Professor of Dermatology and Otology, Department of Veterinary Clinical Sciences, College of Veterinary Medicine, The Ohio State University, Columbus, Ohio

AUTHORS

JOHN GREER CLARK, PhD
Assistant Professor of Audiology, Department of Communication Sciences and Disorders, University of Cincinnati, Cincinnati, Ohio

LYNETTE K. COLE, DVM, MS
Diplomate, American College of Veterinary Dermatology; Associate Professor of Dermatology and Otology, Department of Veterinary Clinical Sciences, College of Veterinary Medicine, The Ohio State University, Columbus, Ohio

LAURENT S. GAROSI, DVM, MRCVS
Diplomate, European College of Veterinary Neurology; RCVS Recognised Specialist in Veterinary Neurology-Head of Neurology, Davies Veterinary Specialists, Higham Gobion, United Kingdom

MARK L. LOWRIE, MA, VetMB, MVM, MRCVS
Diplomate, European College of Veterinary Neurology; RCVS Recognised Specialist in Veterinary Neurology-Head of Neurology, Davies Veterinary Specialists, Higham Gobion, United Kingdom

MARILYN MENOTTI-RAYMOND, PhD
Staff Scientist, Laboratory of Genomic Diversity, Frederick National Laboratory for Cancer Research, National Cancer Institute, Frederick, Maryland

BRADLEY L. NJAA, DVM, MVSc
Diplomate, American College of Veterinary Pathologists, Associate Professor of Veterinary Pathology, Department of Veterinary Pathobiology, Center for Veterinary Health Sciences, Oklahoma State University, Stillwater, Oklahoma

NAOKI OISHI, MD
Visiting Fellow, Kresge Hearing Research Institute, University of Michigan Medical School, Ann Arbor, Michigan; Assistant Professor, Department of Otolaryngology, Keio University School of Medicine, Shinjuku, Tokyo, Japan

DAVID K. RYUGO, PhD
Curran Foundation Chair for Neuroscience, Garvan Institute of Medical Research, Sydney, New South Wales, Australia

JOCHEN SCHACHT, PhD
Professor of Biological Chemistry and Director, Kresge Hearing Research Institute, University of Michigan Medical School, Ann Arbor, Michigan

LESA SCHEIFELE
The Lost Ark, Bethel, Ohio

PETER M. SCHEIFELE, MDr, PhD
Assistant Professor of Audiology and Acoustics, Department of Communication Sciences and Disorders and Neuroaudiology and Neuroanatomy; Department of Medical Education, University of Cincinnati, Cincinnati, Ohio

GEORGE M. STRAIN, PhD
Professor of Neuroscience, Department of Comparative Biomedical Sciences, School of Veterinary Medicine, Louisiana State University, Baton Rouge, Louisiana

MEE JA M. SULA, DVM
Resident, Anatomic Pathology, Department of Veterinary Pathobiology, Center for Veterinary Health Sciences, Oklahoma State University, Stillwater, Oklahoma

NATALIE F. SWINBOURNE, BVM&S, MRCVS
Senior Clinical Training Scholar in Small Animal Surgery, Department of Veterinary Clinical Sciences, Royal Veterinary College, Hatfield, United Kingdom

NATALIE TABACCA, DVM, MS
Veterinary Dermatologist, MedVet Medical and Cancer Center for Pets, Worthington, Ohio

ANDRA E. TALASKA, BS
Research Assistant, Kresge Hearing Research Institute, University of Michigan Medical School, Ann Arbor, Michigan

Contents

Knowledge of the normal structure and function of the canine and feline ear is critical to be able to diagnose abnormalities that either involve the ear or originate within one or more of the ear compartments. In addition, a veterinarian must be aware of various structures within or associated with the ear so that they are not damaged or destroyed while treating an animal with otic disease. This article provides a brief discussion of the various anatomic features of the ear and normal physiology of portions of the ear.

Most veterinary textbooks provide very little guidance regarding ear sampling, processing, and examination. The complexity of the ear, which includes integument, mucosa, cartilage, bone, and neural tissues, and the special procedures required to allow histologic examination are 2 of the more common reasons for reluctance by clinicians and pathologists to thoroughly assess the ear. This article helps demystify both the collection and preparation of ear samples, and briefly describes gross features and key landmarks of the ear. However, it is not the intent to provide an exhaustive account of normal and pathologic findings.

Primary secretory otitis media (PSOM) is a disease that has been described in the Cavalier King Charles spaniel (CKCS). A large, bulging pars flaccida identified on otoscopic examination confirms the diagnosis. However, in many CKCS with PSOM the pars flaccida is flat, and radiographic imaging is needed to confirm the diagnosis. Current treatment for PSOM includes performing a myringotomy into the caudal-ventral quadrant of the pars tensa with subsequent flushing of the mucus out of the bulla using a video otoscope. Repeat myringotomies and flushing of the middle ear are necessary to keep the middle ear free of mucus.

There are four major neuroanatomical structures associated with the ear that, when damaged, result in different neurologic clinical signs. These structures are the facial nerve, the ocular sympathetic tract, the vestibular receptors, and the cochlea. The clinical signs associated with disorders of each structure are discussed, followed by a summary of the diseases that should be considered in each case. The article begins with a description of the neuroanatomy of each of these structures.

Bacterial and fungal otitis constitutes most ear disease in companion animals. However, a wide spectrum of infectious and noninfectious disease processes involve the structures of the ear and are of primary diagnostic consideration in cases of recurrent otitis or those refractive to traditional treatments. This article discusses several common to reasonably rare neoplastic and nonneoplastic space-occupying lesions of the external, middle, and internal ear. Although some conditions present as unique entities, many present similar to or concurrent with otitis, and should be considered in cases of clinically unresponsive otitis.

Cats have among the best hearing of all mammals in that they are extremely sensitive to a broad range of frequencies. The ear is a highly complex structure that is delicately balanced in terms of its biochemistry, types of receptors, ion channels, mechanical properties, and cellular organization. Sensorineural deafness is caused by "flawed" genes that are inherited from one or both parents. Hearing loss can also be acquired as a result of noise trauma from industrialized environment, viral infection, or blunt trauma. To date, it is not practical to intervene and attempt to correct these forms of deafness in cats.

Conductive deafness, caused by outer or middle ear obstruction, may be corrected, whereas sensorineural deafness cannot. Most deafness in dogs is congenital sensorineural hereditary deafness, associated with the genes for white pigment: piebald or merle. The genetic cause has not yet been identified. Dogs with blue eyes have a greater likelihood of hereditary deafness than brown-eyed dogs. Other common forms of sensorineural deafness include presbycusis, ototoxicity, noise-induced hearing loss, otitis interna, and anesthesia. Definitive diagnosis of deafness requires brainstem auditory evoked response testing.

Dog owners and handlers are naturally concerned when suspicion of hearing loss arises for their dogs. Questions frequently asked of the veterinarian center on warning signs of canine hearing loss and what can be done for the dog if hearing loss is confirmed. This article addresses warning signs of canine hearing loss, communication training and safety awareness issues, and the feasibility of hearing aid amplification for dogs.

VETERINARY CLINICS OF NORTH AMERICA: SMALL ANIMAL PRACTICE

RELATED INTEREST

Veterinary Clinics of North America: Exotic Animal Practice
January 2012 (Vol. 15, No. 1)
Mycobacteriosis
Miguel D. Saggese, DVM, MS, PhD, *Guest Editor*

THE CLINICS ARE NOW AVAILABLE ONLINE!
Access your subscription at:
www.theclinics.com

Preface

Otology and Otic Diseases

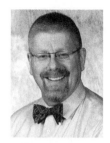 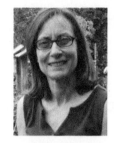

Bradley L. Njaa, DVM,   Lynette K. Cole, DVM,
MVSc, DACVP   MS, DACVD
Guest Editors

It has been 8 years since *Veterinary Clinics of North America: Small Animal Practice* covered the topic of ear diseases. That issue provided a comprehensive review of the normal and diseased ear, incorporating advances in technology with regard to diagnosis of disease, such as endoscopic otoscopes, as well as advanced imaging techniques, including CT and MRI. A majority of the articles focused on external ear disease but few dealt with the other portions of the ear.

Our goal is to provide an issue that is complementary to the previous issue on ear disease with a primary focus on the middle and internal ear. The reader may find the word "internal" to be an unfamiliar term and may be accustomed to the "inner" ear. However, derived from Latin roots, the different compartments of the ear include *auris externa* or external ear, *auris media* or middle ear, and *auris interna* or internal ear.

This issue begins with a brief review of anatomy and physiology of the ear to provide a foundation for the remainder of the issue. Given the paucity of publications that describe pathology of the middle and internal ear, we address this by providing anatomic landmarks and methods for collecting and processing the middle and internal portions of the ear as part of the necropsy exam. This is followed by an article about primary secretory otitis media, a relatively newly described disease that mainly afflicts Cavalier King Charles spaniel dogs and an article on otic masses. Next, there are 5 articles that specifically address conditions of the internal ear beginning with neurological manifestations of ear disease followed by feline deafness, canine deafness, canine hearing loss management, and electrodiagnostic evaluation of auditory function. The final article of this issue is an account of the causes and mechanisms of otoxicity. Where appropriate, glossaries have been included as part of the articles, which are highly specialized or use terminology that may be unfamiliar to most.

We would like to thank Elsevier/Saunders for publishing this issue and John Vassallo for his guidance, support, and patience throughout its development and production. The editors are exceedingly grateful to all of the authors for their dedication and diligence in contributing exceptional articles for this issue. Additionally, Dr Njaa would

Vet Clin Small Anim 42 (2012) ix–x
http://dx.doi.org/10.1016/j.cvsm.2012.08.013
0195-5616/12/$ – see front matter © 2012 Elsevier Inc. All rights reserved.

like to thank his wife, Leanne, and 3 children, Brynne, Layne, and Brooke, for their unending support. Dr Cole would like to thank her husband, Michael Fowler, for his understanding and patience, and pay tribute to her beloved Cavalier King Charles spaniel, "Layla," who passed suddenly on July 1, 2012.

Bradley L. Njaa, DVM, MVSc, DACVP
Department of Veterinary Pathobiology
Center for Veterinary Health Sciences
Oklahoma State University
Stillwater, OK 74078-2007, USA

Lynette K. Cole, DVM, MS, DACVD
Department of Veterinary Clinical Sciences
College of Veterinary Medicine
The Ohio State University
Columbus, OH 43210, USA

E-mail addresses:
brad.njaa@okstate.edu (B.L. Njaa)
Lynette.Cole@cvm.osu.edu (L.K. Cole)

Practical Otic Anatomy and Physiology of the Dog and Cat

Bradley L. Njaa, DVM, MVSc[a],*, Lynette K. Cole, DVM, MS[b],
Natalie Tabacca, DVM, MS[c]

KEYWORDS

- Pinnae • Facial nerve • Chorda tympani • Auditory tube • Tympanic bullae
- Epithelial migration • Auditory ossicles

KEY POINTS

- The close proximity of the auditory ossicles, both the oval and round windows, and both the facial nerve and branch of the facial nerve, the chorda tympani, to the tympanic membrane necessitates the clinician exercise extreme caution when performing myringotomy for the purpose of deep middle ear flushing.
- Bulging of the pars flaccida portion of the tympanic membrane into the external ear canal may be normal in a minority of dogs or may represent a visible sign of otitis externa or primary secretory otitis media.
- Epithelial migration describes the migration of keratinocytes on the external surface of the tympanic membrane away from the stria mallearis onto the surface of the external canal to facilitate cleaning, maintenance of its thinness, and healing.
- The broad tympanic membrane relative to the much smaller footplate of the stapes and the articulated auditory ossicles function to amplify the air pressure wave that vibrates the tympanic membrane to overcome the impedance mismatch between the ambient air (low) and fluid of the membranous labyrinth (high).
- A short segment of the facial canal is devoid of its bony wall near the stapes facilitating insertion of the tendon of the stapedius muscle to the stapes. However, this exposes the facial nerve to the middle ear environment and increases its vulnerability to diseases that may affect the middle ear.

INTRODUCTION

The canine and feline ear can be divided into their component parts, consisting of the pinnae, the external ear canals or external acoustic meatuses, the middle ear, and the internal ear (**Fig. 1**). Knowledge of the normal structure and function of the ear is critical

[a] Department of Veterinary Pathobiology, Center for Veterinary Health Sciences, Oklahoma State University, 226 McElroy Hall, Stillwater, OK 74078-2007, USA; [b] Department of Clinical Sciences, College of Veterinary Medicine, The Ohio State University, 601 Vernon Tharp Street, Columbus, OH 43210, USA; [c] MedVet Medical and Cancer Center for Pets, 300 East Wilson Bridge Road, Wothington, OH 43085, USA
* Corresponding author.
E-mail address: brad.njaa@okstate.edu

Vet Clin Small Anim 42 (2012) 1109–1126
http://dx.doi.org/10.1016/j.cvsm.2012.08.011
0195-5616/12/$ – see front matter © 2012 Elsevier Inc. All rights reserved.

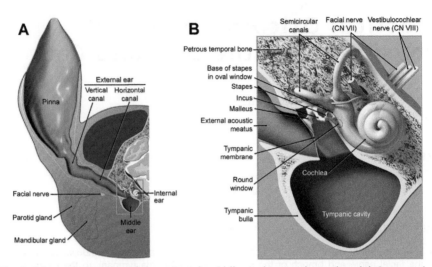

Fig. 1. Schematic diagram of the external, middle, and internal ear, dog. (*A*) Cross-section through the skull. (*B*) Close up view of the middle and internal ear outlined in the blue square in Fig. 1A. (*A and B courtesy of* Dr L.K. Cole and Mr T. Vojt, College of Veterinary Medicine, The Ohio State University, Columbus, OH.)

to be able to diagnose abnormalities that either involve the ear or originate within one or more of the ear compartments. In addition, a veterinarian must be aware of various structures within or associated with the ear so that they are not damaged or destroyed while treating an animal with otic disease. This article provides a brief discussion of the various anatomic features of the ear and normal physiology of portions of the ear. For more in-depth coverage of otic anatomy and physiology, refer to the following references.[1–8]

THE EXTERNAL EAR

The conformation of the pinnae in the dog may be erect or pendulous. Most cats have erect pinnae. Genetic mutations in the cat have affected the development of the pinnae, and resulted in breeds of cats with four ears, folded ears, and curled ears. Cats with the four-eared condition possess a small extra pinna bilaterally, show reduction of the size of their globes, and have a slightly undershot jaw, with a normal body size.[9] Scottish Fold cats are a unique breed with pinnae that are folded. Up to 4 weeks postnatal, Scottish Fold cats have erect pinnae, and then the tips of the ears begin to fold rostrally. All Scottish Fold cats with the folded-ear phenotype, even if heterozygotes, suffer from some degree of osteochondrodysplasia of the distal limbs.[10] The American curl cat breed has pinnae that are curled back at the pinnal apex.

Pinnae play an important role in sound localization and also collect sound waves and transmit them to the tympanic membrane. The pinnae are composed of auricular cartilage that is covered on both sides by haired skin complete with apocrine sweat glands, sebaceous glands, and hair follicles. The convex surface of the pinna has more hair follicles per unit area than the thinner concave surface.[11] The muscles of the pinna are numerous and act to move the ear in specific directions.

The opening of the external ear canal faces dorsolaterally. The quadrangular plate of cartilage, the tragus, forms the lateral boundary of the ear canal. The antitragus is a thin, elongated piece of cartilage caudal to the tragus and separated from it by the intertragic incisure.[1] The intertragic incisure is the anatomic region used to guide the otoscopic cone or otoendoscope into the ear canal for the otoscopic examination (**Fig. 2**). The proximal portion of the auricular cartilage becomes funnel shaped forming the vertical ear canal. The vertical ear canal deviates medially just dorsal to the level of the tympanum to form the horizontal ear canal.[12] There is a prominent cartilaginous ridge that separates the vertical and horizontal ear canals and when the ear is in its normal position, makes otic examination of the horizontal ear canal difficult without elevating this ridge by grasping and lifting the ear pinna (**Fig. 3**). A separate cartilaginous band, the annular cartilage, fits within the base of this conchal tube, giving the external ear canal flexibility. The annular cartilage has fibrous attachments to the osseous external acoustic meatus. The annular cartilage covers the short tubular osseous external acoustic meatus of the tympanic part of the temporal bone. The osseous external acoustic meatus ends at the tympanic annulus.

The dorsorostral margin of the external acoustic meatus is in close apposition to a plateau of bone formed by the zygomatic process of the temporal bone (**Fig. 4**). In most dog breeds, zygomatic process of the temporal bone is short and curved and forms an obtuse angle with the longitudinal axis of the skull. In addition, in most dog breeds, the retroarticular process of the temporomandibular joint is narrow and forms a more obtuse angle relative to the vertical plane. In contrast, some dogs, such as pit bull terriers, have a longer and broader zygomatic process of the temporal bone that forms a right angle or slightly acute angle to the longitudinal axis. The retroarticular process is much broader and longer and forms a much more acute angle

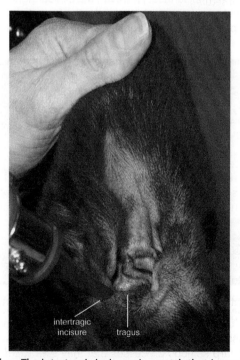

Fig. 2. Right pinna, dog. The intertragic incisures is a notch that is caudal to the tragus and represents a useful anatomic region for insertion of an otoscopic cone (shown) or otoendoscope into the ear canal for the otoscopic examination. (*Courtesy of* Dr L.K. Cole and Mr J. Harvey, College of Veterinary Medicine, The Ohio State University, Columbus, OH.)

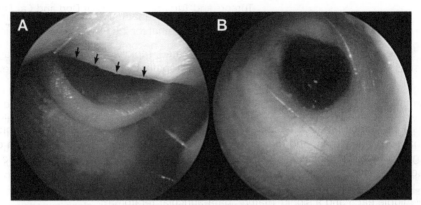

Fig. 3. Ear canal, dog. (*A*) Video otoscopic image, junction of vertical and horizontal canal. A prominent cartilaginous ridge (*arrows*) is visible and represents a landmark that separates the vertical and horizontal ear canals. (*B*) Video otoscopic image, horizontal canal. This represents the view down the horizontal ear canal after elevating the prominent cartilaginous ridge by grasping and lifting the ear pinna. (*Courtesy of* Dr L.K. Cole, College of Veterinary Medicine, The Ohio State University, Columbus, OH.)

relative to the vertical plane (see **Fig. 4**). In aggregate, these variations in pit bull terriers result in an external acoustic meatus that is deeper and possibly better protected relative to the external surface. However, the clinical significance of this deeper location and more acute angles can inhibit the depth of insertion of the otoendoscope when attempting to perform a myringotomy using the video otoscope.

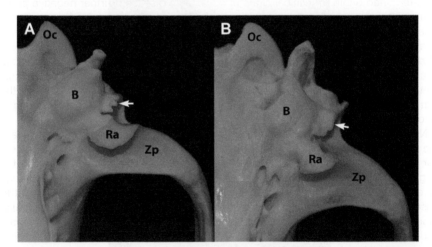

Fig. 4. External ear, dog. (*A*) Macerated skull, pit bull. The external acoustic meatus (*arrow*) opens into an area that is made shallow by a broad retroarticular process (Ra) and a longer zygomatic process of the temporal bone (Zp). The angle that is formed by the plateau of bone approximates 90 degrees or slightly less. (*B*) Macerated skull, shepherd cross dog. The external acoustic meatus (*arrow*) opens into an area that is more open with a small, shallower retroarticular process (Ra) and a shorter zygomatic process of the temporal bone (Zp). In this dog, the angle formed is more obtuse providing greater access to the ear by otoscopic examination. B, tympanic bulla; Oc, occipital condyles. (*Courtesy of* Dr B.L. Njaa, Center for Veterinary Health Sciences, Oklahoma State University, Stillwater, OK.)

The epidermis lining the external ear canal is similar histologically to the pinna; however, in most breeds, hairs are fewer and do not extend the length of the ear canal.[13] A very few fine hairs are found distal to the tympanic membrane. These hairs are a useful landmark when flushing an ear to locate the tympanic membrane in an abnormal ear (**Fig. 5**). Cocker spaniel dogs typically have excessive compound hair follicles in the horizontal ear canal compared with sparsely distributed, simple hair follicles in greyhound dogs and mixed breed dogs.[14]

The external ear canal also contains sebaceous glands and ceruminous glands, which are modified apocrine glands. Cerumen is an emulsion that coats the ear canal. It is composed of desquamated keratinized squamous epithelial cells along with the secretions from the sebaceous and ceruminous glands of the ears. The dermis of the external ear canal is typical, consisting of collagen and elastic fibers and a subcutaneous layer that separates the dermis from the deeper cartilage layer.[1]

The external ear and external canal terminate medially at the tympanic membrane. It is important to note that the tympanic membrane is orientated at a 45-degree angle relative to the central axis of the horizontal external acoustic meatus. In some breeds, the tympanic membrane is also variably orientated rostrally.[8] From a clinical perspective, this angle can be used to advantage while performing a deep external ear flush, allowing one to be able to pass a catheter along the ventral floor of the horizontal ear canal without rupturing the tympanic membrane to remove all the flushing solution and saline (**Fig. 6**).

THE TYMPANIC MEMBRANE

The tympanic membrane is a semitransparent three-layer membrane. The tympanic membrane is divided into two sections: the smaller dorsal pars flaccida and the larger ventral pars tensa. In most dogs and in the cat the pars flaccida is flat. If the pars flaccida bulges laterally, this is an uncommon finding in normal dogs but may also be found in ears of dogs with otitis externa (**Fig. 7**). Histologic differences have not been identified between flat and bulging pars flaccidas in normal dogs, so it seems unlikely that a structural difference explains a bulging pars flaccida.[15] However, in

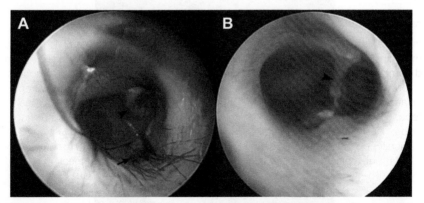

Fig. 5. Video otoscopic image of the tympanic membrane. (*A*) Tympanic membrane, right ear, dog. A prominent tuft of hair is immediately distal to the tympanic membrane (*arrow*). In the dog, the stria mallearis is distinctly "C"-shaped stria malleris (*arrowhead*). (*B*) Tympanic membrane, right ear, cat. The stria mallearis in cats is much more straightened and perpendicular (*arrowhead*), lacking the "C"-shape observed dogs. (*Courtesy of* Dr L.K. Cole, College of Veterinary Medicine, The Ohio State University, Columbus, OH.)

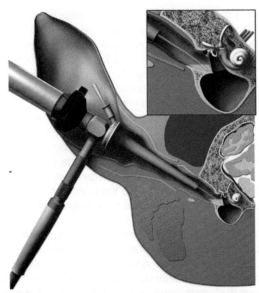

Fig. 6. Schematic diagram illustrating placement of the otoendoscope in the ear canal while performing a deep ear flush of the external ear canal. Inset diagram is a higher magnification depicting the typical 45-degree angle of the tympanic membrane and a catheter passing ventrally to suction the flushing solution and saline from the external ear canal. (*Courtesy of* Dr L.K. Cole and Mr T. Vojt, College of Veterinary Medicine, The Ohio State University, Columbus, OH.)

Cavalier King Charles spaniel dogs, a bulging pars flaccida is indicative of primary secretory otitis media, a disease in which mucus fills the middle ear cavity, possibly as a result of auditory tube dysfunction (please refer the article by Dr Cole elsewhere in this issue).[16]

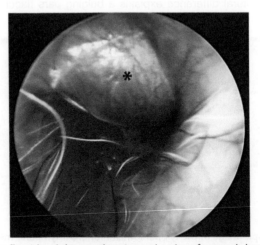

Fig. 7. Bulging pars flaccida, right ear, dog. In a minority of normal dogs, the pars flaccida bulges (*asterisk*) into the external ear canal. However, a bulging pars flaccida may be seen in dogs with otitis externa or in Cavalier King Charles spaniel dogs with primary secretory otitis media. (*Courtesy of* Dr L.K. Cole, College of Veterinary Medicine, The Ohio State University, Columbus, OH.)

The pars tensa comprises most of the total surface area of the tympanic membrane. It is very thin but extremely tough and robuse, with radiating ridges. The manubrium of the malleus is embedded in the tympanic membrane of the pars tensa with its flattened surface facing craniolaterally, and its medial contours bulging from the medial surface of the tympanic membrane into middle ear compartment. The pars tensa has a concave shape when viewed externally because of the tension applied to the internal surface of the membrane, where the manubrium of the malleus is attached. The point of greatest depression, opposite the distal end of the manubrium, is called the umbo (**Fig. 8**).[1,6,7]

The outline of the manubrium of the malleus, the stria mallearis, may be visualized when the tympanic membrane is viewed externally. The stria mallearis is hook- or C-shaped in the dog, with the concave aspect of the "C" facing rostrally (see **Fig. 5A**). In the cat, the stria mallearis is straight with no hook- or C-shape (see **Fig. 5B**). Based on a study of experimentally ruptured normal tympanic membranes, if one performs a myringotomy, the membrane should regenerate by Day 14, with complete healing between 21 and 35 days.[17]

A unique feature of the tympanic membrane is its ability to remain extremely thin and resilient despite the continuous secretions of dermal adnexal glands. The maintenance of its thinness and self-cleaning function of the external ear is primarily achieved by a process called "epithelial migration."

Epithelial migration is the movement of keratinocytes of the lateral (external auditory canal) surface of the tympanic membrane and of the auditory canal epithelium. It provides a self-cleaning mechanism for removal of debris from the external auditory canal and tympanic membrane. During this process, cerumen is transported away from the tympanic membrane and toward the opening of the distal auditory canal. This prevents the accumulation of cerumen that could lead to conductive hearing loss.[18–21]

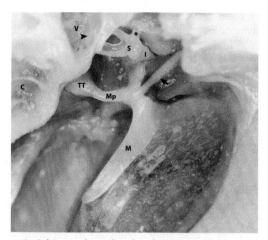

Fig. 8. Chorda tympani, right ear, dog. The chorda tympani (*arrow*) courses dorsally across the neck of the malleus ventral to the muscular process of the malleus (Mp), in close proximity to the pars tensa. The stapes (S) is anchored in the oval or vestibular window and the foot plate (*arrowhead*) is clearly visible in the opened vestibule (V). The stapes and incus (I) articulate to form the incudostapedius joint. Tendon of the stapedius muscle (*asterisk*). C, cochlea; M, manubrium of the malleus; TT, tensor tympani muscle. (*Courtesy of* Dr B.L. Njaa, Center for Veterinary Health Sciences, Oklahoma State University, Stillwater, OK.)

Epithelial migration maintains the tympanic membrane as thin and highly responsive by transporting stratum corneum keratinocytes off of the tympanic membrane toward the open end of the external auditory canal.[18,21–23] This stratum corneal keratinocyte migration along the surface of the tympanic membrane also serves to repair punctures, whether they are spontaneous perforations[24–28] or postoperative incisions (myringotomy sites).[29]

The epithelial migration rate and pattern has now been described for normal tympanic membranes in many species including humans,[27,29–36] gerbils,[20,37] rats,[38] and guinea pigs.[20,39–42] Unfortunately, epithelial migration information is not available for normal feline tympanic membranes. However, epithelial migration of canine tympanic membranes has been investigated.[43] Waterproof ink markers were placed on two sites of the pars tensa, caudal to the stria mallearis, and one on the center of the pars flaccida of tympanic membranes of normal laboratory dogs. Each inked membrane was evaluated four times, every 6 to 8 days using video otoscopy and a digital capture system. Image processing software was used to analyze the migration pattern and calculate the epithelial migration rate in microns per day. The direction of movement for each ink drop was recorded as outward (toward the periphery of the tympanic membrane and external auditory canal) or inward (toward the center of the tympanic membrane) and the overall pattern for each ink drop on each dog's membrane was recorded.

The mean overall epithelial migration rate for ink drops placed on the pars tensa and pars flaccida was 96.4 and 225.4 um/d, respectively. All ink drops were observed to migrate outward, toward the periphery of the tympanic membrane and external auditory canal. Ink drops never migrated from the pars tensa onto the pars flaccida or vice versa. A percentage of the ink drops at all three locations were observed to migrate off of the tympanic membrane and onto the epithelium of the external auditory canal. Migration off of the tympanic membrane by the last evaluation day was noted most frequently for the pars flaccida location. Most of the ink drops (90.6%) moved in a radial direction, in a straight line outward like spokes on a bicycle wheel. The remaining ink drops moved in a centrifugal pattern, in which the ink drops took a curved course outward from the original location.[43]

Functionally, the tympanic membrane vibrates in response to sound-generated air pressure waves, which translates into fluid pressure waves in the aqua environment of the internal ear compartments of the membranous labyrinth. However, air and fluid have very different impedance (the tendency of a medium to oppose movement brought about by a pressure wave).[44] Because fluid has higher impedance than air, a direct transfer of a pressure wave from air to water is insufficient to move through the internal ear fluid compartment. This is referred to as "impedance mismatch." Thus, the middle ear functions as an impedance-matching device by the following mechanisms. First, the surface area of the tympanic membrane is much larger than the surface area of the foot plate of the stapes anchored in the vestibular or oval window of the petrous portion of the temporal bone. Second, the incus and malleus act as a lever system. In aggregate, these two features inherent of the middle ear function to amplify the pressure wave and overcome the impedance mismatch.[44] From a clinical perspective, a perforation of the tympanic membrane, articular defect to the auditory ossicles, or altered middle ear function because of otitis media may contribute to impairing of this impedance mismatch, and thus result in impaired detection of sound.

THE MIDDLE EAR

The middle ear is an air-filled alcove fortified on nearly every fringe by bone; laterally by the tympanic portion of the temporal bone and medial surface of the tympanic membrane; ventrally by the tympanic bulla; medially by the petrous portion of the temporal bone; and dorsally by petrous portion and the tympanic portion of the temporal bone (**Fig. 9**).[1–3] Rostrally, this chamber is open to the nasopharynx by the narrow musculotubular canal, through which penetrates the cartilage conduit of the auditory tube and the tensor veli palatine muscle.[4] Finally, three auditory ossicles (malleus, incus, and stapes) form a chain of bones dorsally in the middle ear and provide a direct bony connection between the aerated external environment and the fluid environment of the perilymph of the internal ear.[1,4]

The mean middle ear cavity volume of mesaticephalic dogs as measured by computed tomography technique is 1.5 mL, and the middle ear cavity volume increases in a nonlinear fashion by body weight[45] suggesting that on average when flushing the middle ear cavity during a deep ear flush or when instilling medications into the tympanic bulla that 1.5 mL should be a sufficient volume in an average-size dog.

The tympanic cavity is divided into the epitympanic recess, the tympanic cavity proper, and the ventral cavity. The epitympanic recess is the smallest of the three areas and is occupied almost entirely by the head of the malleus and incus (see **Fig. 9**).[1,12] The tympanic cavity proper is adjacent to the tympanic membrane. On the medial wall of the tympanic cavity proper, there is a bony eminence, the promontory of the petrous portion of the temporal bone, which houses the cochlea. The

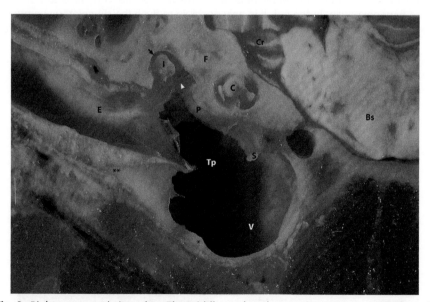

Fig. 9. Right ear, rostral view, dog. The middle ear has three main compartments. The epitympanic recess (*arrow*) is the smallest, most dorsal compartment occupied by the articulated malleus and incus (I). The next largest is the tympanic cavity proper (Tp) demarcated laterally by the tympanic membrane (torn in this image) and medially by the promontory of the petrous portion of the temporal bone (P). The largest is the ventral compartment (V) surrounded by the bone of the tympanic bulla (*asterisk*). Ventral bony ridge of the external acoustic meatus (*double asterisk*); stapes (*arrowhead*). Bs, brainstem; C, cochlea; Cr, cerebellar cortex; E, external ear canal; F, facial nerve in its facial canal; S, incomplete septum bulla. (*Courtesy of* Dr B.L. Njaa, Center for Veterinary Health Sciences, Oklahoma State University, Stillwater, OK.)

promontory is located opposite to the mid-dorsal aspect of the tympanic membrane. The cochlear (round) window is located in the caudolateral portion of the promontory[6,12] and is covered by a thin membrane.[6] The vestibular (oval) window is located on the dorsolateral surface of the promontory, medial to the pars flaccida.[1,12] Normally, the stapes is firmly lodged in the vestibular window with its baseplate held in place by the annular ligament of the vestibular window. The largest of the three cavities is the ventral cavity, occupying the ventromedial portion of the tympanic bulla (see **Fig. 9**).[1,2]

Within the middle ear of the dog and cat is a bony septum referred to as the septum bulla (**Fig. 10**).[1–4] In the dog, the bulla septum is a small, incomplete ridge that only makes contact with the petrous portion of the temporal bone rostrally and often has tiny, elongate bony spicules with bulbous ends.[1,8] In the cat, the septum bulla abuts the petrous portion of the temporal bone and separates the tympanic cavity into two compartments: the dorsolateral epitympanic cavity (pars tympanica) and the ventromedial tympanic cavity (pars endotympanica).[1,4,8] This separation is almost complete, allowing communication between the two compartments only through two small openings: one is between the septum bulla and petrous portion of the temporal bone and the other is located caudally, just lateral to the round window. The difference in the size of this septum between the dog and the cat is of clinical significance in the treatment and management of middle ear disease. Because the bulla septum is very small in the dog, resulting in a large opening between the tympanic cavity proper and the ventral bulla, this allows one to be able to flush the entire tympanic bulla. In the cat, it is only possible to flush the dorsolateral compartment of the tympanic bulla because it is divided into two compartments. Therefore,

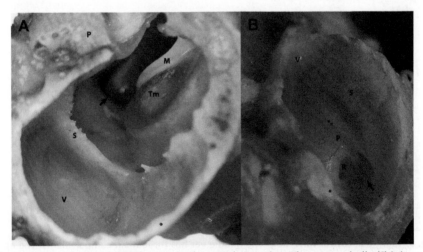

Fig. 10. Septum bullae. (*A*) Right ear, caudoventral view, dog. The septum bulla (S) is incomplete separating the tympanic cavity proper from the ventral tympanic cavity (V). Dorsorostrally, the auditory tube is visible (*arrow*). Tympanic bulla (*asterisk*). M, manubrium of the malleus; P, petrous portion of the temporal bone; Tm, tympanic membrane. (*B*) Left ear, ventral view, cat. The septum bulla (S) is complete and abuts (*double asterisk*) the petrous portion of the temporal bone (P). Caudally, there is an open communication (*arrow*) between the two cavities formed by the septum bulla. Tympanic bulla (*asterisk*). R, round window; V, ventral tympanic cavity. (*Courtesy of* Dr B.L. Njaa, Center for Veterinary Health Sciences, Oklahoma State University, Stillwater, OK.)

in most cases of middle ear disease in the cat, surgical management of the ear disease is necessary. In addition, one needs to avoid the use of ointment-based medications or otic packing material instilled into the ear of the cat with a ruptured tympanic membrane, because the medication may leak into the large ventromedial compartment and become trapped.

AUDITORY OSSICLES

The auditory ossicular chain formed by articulations between the malleus and incus, or the incudomallearis joint, and the incus and the stapes, or the incudostapedius joint, functions as a lever system. In concert with the marked difference in surface area between the tympanic membrane and the footplate of the stapes, the net result is amplification of the initial air pressure wave to account for the increase impedance of the fluid in the membranous labyrinthine compartment of the cochlear of the internal ear.[44]

The malleus, the largest of the auditory ossicles, has a long process, the manubrium, embedded in the tympanic membrane. Projecting rostrally from the neck of the malleus is the muscular process, the attachment site for the tensor tympani muscle. Dorsally, the head of the malleus and body of the incus articulate to form the incudomallearis joint, anchored in the epitympanic recess by ligaments. A small branch of the facial nerve, the chorda tympani, exits the facial canal, passes beneath the base of the muscular process of the malleus medial to but in close proximity to the pars flaccida before exiting the middle ear (see **Fig. 8**).[1,2,4] Once beyond the ear, the chorda tympani merges with the lingual branch of the mandibular nerve (cranial nerve V) once exiting through a canal in the rostrodorsal wall of the tympanic bulla to innervate the rostral third of the tongue.[1] Otitis media and traumatic or surgical rupture dorsal in the tympanic membrane can potentially result in impairment of taste.

The incus is much smaller that the malleus with two bony extensions or crura (**Fig. 11**). Although the short crus is largely anchored in the epitympanic recess along with the incudomallearis joint, the long crus extends medially and caudally from the malleus to articulate with the stapes (see **Fig. 8**).[1,2,8] At the distal, medial end of the long crus is a small flat bone, the lenticular process, that articulates with the head of the stapes to form the incudostapedius joint (shown in Figs. 1 and 3 in the article by Garosi elsewhere in this issue).[1,2,4,8]

The smallest of the auditory ossicles, the stapes, is a triangular bone that is anchored in the oval or vestibular window by its annular ligament (see **Figs. 8** and **11**). It functions as a piston that transduces tympanic membrane vibrations to fluid waves in the perilymph of the internal ear membranous labyrinthine compartments.[1,2,8]

The facial nerve enters the internal acoustic meatus and travels through the facial canal of the petrous portion of the temporal bone, exiting the skull through the stylomastoid foramen immediately caudal to the external acoustic meatus.[1-3,8] The facial canal is a bony tunnel that courses through the petrous portion of the temporal bone. In a small region caudal and dorsal to the caudal crus of the stapes, this bony canal is incomplete and exposed to the middle ear compartment. The opening corresponds to the region where the tendon of the stapedius muscle emerges and inserts near the head of the stapes (**Fig. 12**; also shown in Fig. 1 in the article by Garosi elsewhere in this issue). This opening also corresponds to the location where otitis media can infiltrate through connective tissue and result in facial neuritis. Otitis media resulting in facial nerve paralysis causes facial drooping or spasms and ocular signs. If the patient develops a head tilt, this is a clinical indication of vestibulocochlear nerve involvement caused by an ascending otitis interna (see the article by Garosi elsewhere in this issue).

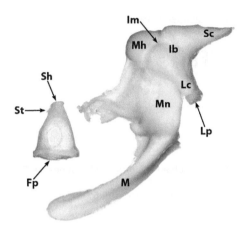

Fig. 11. Auditory ossicles, right ear, dog. The stapes is the smallest bone with a narrow head (Sh), a broader foot plate (Fp), and an attachment site close to the head for the tendon of the stapedius muscle. The malleus and incus are articulated to form the incudomallearis joint (Im). The malleus has a long manubrium (M) That is embedded in the tympanic membrane, a neck (Mn), and head (Mh). The incus has a body (Ib), short crus (Sc), and long crus (Lc). At the end of the long crus is the lenticular process (Lp) that articulates with the head of the stapes to form the incudostapedius joint. Insertion site for tendon of stapedius muscle (St). (*Courtesy of* Dr B.L. Njaa, Center for Veterinary Health Sciences, Oklahoma State University, Stillwater, OK.)

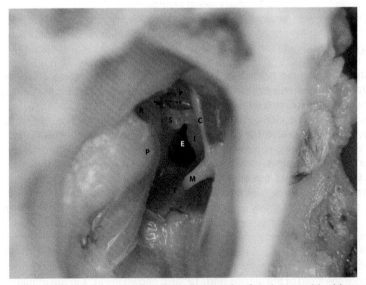

Fig. 12. Right middle ear, dog. In this ventral view, the facial nerve (*double asterisk*) is exposed caudal to the stapes (S) with an incomplete bony ridge of the facial canal (*arrowhead*) visible dorsally. The tendon of the stapedius muscle (*arrow*) emerges from the same opening in the facial canal. C, chorda tympani; E, epitympanic recess; I, incus; M, muscular process of the malleus; P, promontory; R, round window; T, tensor tympani muscle. (*Courtesy of* Dr B.L. Njaa, DVM, MVSc, Center for Veterinary Health Sciences, Oklahoma State University, Stillwater, OK.)

THE AUDITORY TUBE

The auditory tube is a short canal that extends from the nasopharynx to the rostral portion of the tympanic cavity proper (**Fig. 13**). It functions to equalize pressure on both sides of the tympanic membrane.[46] The auditory tube is divided into three portions: (1) cartilaginous (proximal and opens into the nasopharyx); (2) junctional (part of tube at which the cartilaginous and osseous portions connect); and (3) the osseous potion (distal and opens into the rostral middle ear). The osseous portion of the auditory tube is patent at all times, whereas the cartilaginous portion is closed at rest and opens during swallowing.[47]

Contraction of the levator muscle and tensor palatini muscle function in concert to open the auditory tube. The entrance to the auditory tube is obscured behind the soft palate, midway between the caudal aspect of the nares and the caudal border of the soft palate.[12] Based on contrast-enhanced computed tomographic imaging, the auditory tube originates from the rostral, dorsomedial aspect of the bulla and enters the dorsolateral aspect of the nasopharynx just caudal to the hamulus process of the pterygoid bone.[48]

THE INTERNAL EAR

The petrous portion of the temporal bone is the densest bone in the body, forming the medial margin of the middle ear. It is an angular, conical bone with its apex pointed rostral and ventral (**Fig. 14**). Relative to other bones of the skull, the petrous portion of the temporal bone is more yellow and does not contain medullary or marrow compartments. A bony bulge that protrudes lateral and ventral from the petrous temporal bone is referred to as the "promontory."[1,2,8] The basal turn of the cochlea is demarcated by this promontory. The vestibular or oval window and cochlear or round window flank the promontory on opposing sites. Rostrally, a second bulge is present in dogs and cats, denoting the cochlea. Contrary to many textbook diagrams that clearly delineate the membranous labyrinthine

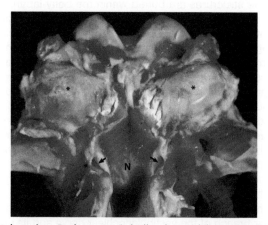

Fig. 13. Auditory tubes, dog. Both tympanic bullae (*asterisks*) are exposed after removal of the mandible and associated muscles. Bilaterally opening into the nasopharynx (N) are the auditory tubes (*arrows*). Sutures were placed and used to hold the auditory tubes open. However, they are typically closed. (*Courtesy of* Dr B.L. Njaa, Center for Veterinary Health Sciences, Oklahoma State University, Stillwater, OK.)

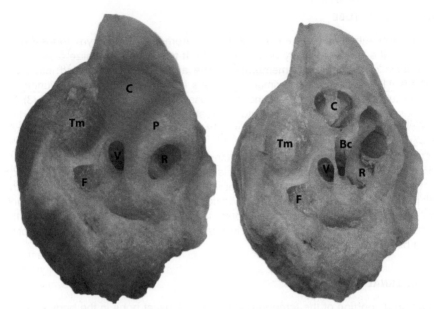

Fig. 14. Petrous portion of the temporal bone, left ear, cat. The bone on the right has had the cochlea and promontory opened with the use of bone cutters. The most prominent medial bulge is the promontory (P), flanked by the vestibular or oval window (V), and the cochlear or round window (R). This promontory corresponds to the basal turn of the cochlea (Bc). A rostral bulge corresponds to the spiral cochlea (C). A bony depression (Tm) is the fossa for the tensor tympani muscle. The facial canal (F) is partially opened in these sections. (*Courtesy of* Dr B.L. Njaa, Center for Veterinary Health Sciences, Oklahoma State University, Stillwater, OK.)

spiraled cochlea, bulging saccule and utricle, and looping semicircular canals, in reality these delicate structures are buried within the bony labyrinth of the petrous portion of the temporal bone and are not clearly visible without sophisticated imaging equipment.

When performing a myringotomy during a deep ear flush, it is important to avoid damaging the promontory and the round and oval windows so as to not induce iatrogenic neurologic complications. It is also important to avoid damaging the ossicles, which are important for the amplification and transmission of sound waves to the internal ear. Because the oval and round windows are located on the dorsal and caudal aspect of the promontory, respectively, the promontory is located opposite to the mid-dorsal aspect of the tympanic membrane, and the ossicles are located dorsorostrally, the myringotomy should be performed in the caudoventral quadrant of the tympanic membrane.

The two main functional units of the internal ear are the auditory system and the vestibular system.[44] The former provides a sense of hearing; the latter a sense of balance. The internal ear portion of the auditory system comprises the cochlea and associated cochlear branch of the vestibulocochlear nerve and its connections to the central nervous system. The vestibular system comprises several fluid-filled, epithelial-lined compartments (saccule, utricle, and semicircular canals), which continually provide input to the brain regarding head and body orientation and direction and speed of movement.

THE COCHLEA

The cochlea is the highly coiled series of fluid-filled compartments. The two main compartments include the scala vestibuli and the scala tympani, both containing peri-lymph, a distillate of cerebrospinal fluid. At the apex of the cochlea both scala are in direct communication by the helicotrema.[1,2,4,49,50] Sandwiched between these two scala is the much smaller fluid-filled scala media or cochlear duct (shown in the articles by Ryugo and Strain elsewhere in this issue). The scala media is separated from the scala vestibuli by the vestibular membrane (Reissner's membrane) and from the scala tympani by the basilar membrane (shown in the article by Ryugo elsewhere in this issue). These three compartments spiral 2.5 turns about a central axis known as the "modiolus," through which runs the cochlear nerve.[1,2,4,49,50]

Atop the basilar membrane is the organ of Corti, the sensory or spiral organ of hearing. The sensory cells are called hair cells, denoted as inner hair cells and outer hair cells, relative to a central modiolus point of reference. A gelatinous, collagen-containing tectorial membrane is suspended over the organ of Corti, in which hair cells are apically embedded. The hair cells receive afferent and efferent innervation from the cochlear branch of the vestibulocochlear nerve (cranial nerve VIII).[44,49,50]

Hair cells are not neurons but are cellular mechanoreceptors with apical sensory "hairs" that are not pilosebaceous units but highly specialized stereocilia and kinocilia. Fluid pressure waves in the scala vestibuli from vibrations from the stapes result in deflection of the basilar membrane of the scala media. This results in movement of the organ of Corti and the tectorial membrane perched on the apical cilia of hair cells causes them to bend. The direction these apical cilia bend determines if the cell becomes depolarized or hyperpolarized. Depolarized hair cells release neurotrans-mitter across its basolateral margin at synapses with neurons of the cochlear nerve, whereas hyperpolarization of the cell inhibits neurotransmitter release. Along its length, the basilar membrane varies from narrow and thick to wide and thin, thereby enabling detection of various frequencies along its entire length (shown in the article by Ryugo elsewhere in this issue).[44,49,50]

The auditory system is covered in much greater depth in several articles in this issue.

THE VESTIBULAR SYSTEM

The caudal half to one-third of the petrous portion of the temporal bone contains the vestibular structures, including the saccule, the utricle, and the semicircular canals (shown in the article by Ryugo elsewhere in this issue).[1–4,8,49,50] The saccule and utricle are located within the vestibule in close proximity to the stapes and basal turn of the cochlea. Neurosensory epithelial hair cells aggregate in a thickened region of the wall of these endolymph-filled cavities called the macula. The saccular macula is oriented vertically, whereas the uticular macula is oriented horizontally. Overlying each maculae is a gelatinous layer of polysaccharide to which are adhered small calcium carbonate crystals called "otoliths." Because these otoliths have greater density than endolymph, as the head moves, otoliths under the pull of gravity cause the apical cilia of hair cells to become deflected. In aggregate, the maculae of the utricle and saccule function to detect the steady tilt of the head.[44]

Semicircular canals branch caudally from the utricle in orthogonal planes. Each canal bulges at its direct connection to the utricle called "ampullae." Specialized neurosen-sory structures within the ampullae are called "crista ampularis," which contain sensory hair cells. Apical cilia from these hair cells are embedded in a gelatinous structure called the cupula. Movement of these cupula relative to their embedded hair cells is how rapid angular acceleration of an animal's head is detected.[44,49,50]

Vestibular function and dysfunction is covered more extensively elsewhere in this issue.

SUMMARY

The ear is often thought of as pinnae and associated structures. The pinnae and associated dermis is a direct extension of the epidermis and dermis of the body and may be a predilection site for various dermatologic entities. The middle ear is a bony encased, air-filled chamber whose only connection to ambient air is through the auditory tube. Within this cavity are three crucial bones, the auditory ossicles, which transduce air pressure changes in the tympanic membrane to fluid waves in the internal ear acting as an impedance matching device. Specialized neurosensory epithelium within the cochlear portion of the membranous labyrinth of the internal ear convert these fluid waves into action potentials that are transmitted to the brain by the cochlear nerve for recognition as sound. Variation in the width and density of the basilar membrane of the scala media mediates variable recognition of various sound frequencies. Similar neurosensory epithelium in the vestibular portions of the internal ear similarly respond to steady and rapid acceleration movements of the head to maintain balance and normal proprioception by signals traveling through the vestibular branch of the vestibulocochlear nerve. Therefore, numerous loci within this complex sensory organ can become dysfunctional. Recognition of clinical disease necessitates a "sound" understanding of otic anatomy and physiology and keen observation skills.

REFERENCES

1. Evans HE, de Lahunta A. The ear. In: Evans HE, de Lahunta A, editors. Miller's anatomy of the dog. 4th edition. St. Louis (MO): Elsevier; 2013. p. 731–45.
2. Liebich HG, Konig HE. Vestibulocochlear organ. In: Konig HE, Liebich HG, editors. Veterinary anatomy of domestic animals: textbook and colour atlas. 3rd edition. New York: Schattauer; 2007. p. 593–608.
3. Boyd JS. A color atlas of clinical anatomy of the dog & cat. Aylesbury, bucks (England): Mosby-Wolfe; 1995.
4. Constantinescu GM, Schaller O, editors. Illustrated veterinary anatomical nomenclature. 3rd edition. Stuttgart (Germany): Enke Verlag; 2012.
5. Cole LK. Anatomy and physiology of the canine ear. Vet Dermatol 2009;20: 412–21.
6. Kumar A. Anatomy of the canine and feline ear. In: Gotthelf LN, editor. Small animal ear diseases. 2nd edition. St. Louis (MO): Elsevier Saunders; 2005. p. 1–21.
7. Heine PA. Anatomy of the ear. Vet Clin North Am Small Anim Pract 2004;34: 379–95.
8. Njaa BL. The ear. In: Zachary JF, McGavin MD, editors. Pathologic basis of veterinary disease. 5th edition. St. Louis (MO): Elsevier Mosby; 2012. p. 1153–93.
9. Little CC. Four-ears, a recessive mutation in the cat. J Hered 1957;48(2):57.
10. Takanosu M, Takanosu T, Suzuki H, et al. Incomplete dominant osteochondrodysplasia in heterozygous Scottish fold cats. J Small Anim Pract 2008;49:197–9.
11. Calhoun ML, Stinson AW. Integument. In: Dellmann HD, Brown EM, editors. Textbook of veterinary histology. 3rd edition. Philadelphia: Lea & Febiger; 1987. p. 382–415.
12. Harvey RG, Harari J, Delauche AJ. The normal ear. Ear diseases of the dog and cat. Ames (IA): Iowa State University Press; 2001. 9–41.
13. Fraser G. The histopathology of the external auditory meatus of the dog. J Comp Pathol 1961;71:253–60.

14. Stout-Graham M, Kainer RA, Whalen LR, et al. Morphologic measurements of the external horizontal ear canal of dogs. Am J Vet Res 1990;51:990–4.
15. Cole LK, Weisbrode SE, Smeak DD. Variation in gross and histological appearance of the canine pars flaccida. Vet Dermatol 2007;18:464–8.
16. Stern-Bertholtz W, Sjostrom L, Hakanson NW. Primary secretory otitis media in the cavalier King Charles spaniel: a review of 61 cases. J Small Anim Pract 2003;44: 253–6.
17. Steiss JE, Boosinger TR, Wright JC, et al. Healing of experimentally perforated tympanic membranes, demonstrated by electrodiagnostic testing and histopathology. J Am Anim Hosp Assoc 1992;28:307–10.
18. Jahn AF, Santos-Sacchi J. Physiology of the ear. 2nd edition. San Diego (CA): Singular/Thomson Learning; 2001. 689.
19. Logas DB. Diseases of the ear canal. Vet Clin North Am Small Anim Pract 1994; 24:905–19.
20. Tinling SP, Chole RA. Gerbilline cholesteatoma development part I: epithelial migration pattern and rate on the gerbil tympanic membrane: comparisons with human and guinea pig. Otolaryngol Head Neck Surg 2006;134(5):788–93.
21. Litton WB. Epidermal migration in the ear: the location and characteristics of the generati center revealed by utilizing a radioactive desoxyribose nucleic acid precursor. Acta Otolaryngol 1968;66(Suppl 240):5–39.
22. Lim DJ. Structure and function of the tympanic membrane: a review. Acta Otorhinolaryngol Belg 1995;49(2):101–15.
23. White PD. Medical management of chronic otitis in dogs. Compend Contin Educ Pract Vet 1999;21(8):716–28.
24. Clawson JP, Litton WB. The healing process of tympanic membrane perforations. Trans Am Acad Ophthalmol Otolaryngol 1971;75(6):1302–12.
25. Johnson A, Hawke M. The function of migratory epidermis in the healing of tympanic membrane perforations in guinea-pig. A photographic study. Acta Otolaryngol 1987;103(1–2):81–6.
26. Wang WQ, Wang ZM, Chi FL. Spontaneous healing of various tympanic membrane perforations in the rat. Acta Otolaryngol 2004;124(10):1141–4.
27. Simmons FB. Epithelial migration in central-type tympanic perforations. Preliminary report on a potential diagnostic tool. Arch Otolaryngol 1961;74:435–6.
28. McIntire C, Benitez JT. Spontaneous repair of the tympanic membrane. histpathological studies in the cat. Ann Otol Rhinol Laryngol 1970;79(6):1129–31.
29. Deong KK, Prepageran N, Raman R. Epithelial migration of the postmyringoplasty tympanic membrane. Otol Neurotol 2006;27(6):855–8.
30. Alberti PW. Epithelial migration on the tympanic membrane. J Laryngol Otol 1964; 78:808–30.
31. Michaels L, Soucek S. Auditory epithelial migration on the human tympanic membrane .2. The existence of 2 discrete migratory pathways and their embryologic correlates. Am J Anat 1990;189(3):189–200.
32. Makino K, Amatsu M. Epithelial migration on the tympanic membrane and external canal. Arch Otorhinolaryngol 1986;243(1):39–42.
33. Bonding P, Charabi S. Epithelial migration in mastoid cavities. Clin Otolaryngol 1994;19(4):306–9.
34. Bahadur S, Kacker SK. Epithelial migration in posterosuperior retraction pockets and in grafted tympanic membranes. Ear Nose Throat J 1982;61(2):98–101.
35. Moriarty BG, Johnson AP, Patel P. Patterns of epithelial migration in the unaffected ear in patients with a history of unilateral cholesteatoma. Clin Otolaryngol Allied Sci 1991;16(1):48–51.

36. Tang IP, Prepageran N, Raman R, et al. Epithelial migration in the atelectatic tympanic membrane. J Laryngol Otol 2009;123(12):1321–4.
37. Yi ZX, Shi GS, Huang CC. Age-related epithelial migration on the tympanic membrane of the Mongolian gerbil. Otolaryngol Head Neck Surg 1988;98(6): 564–7.
38. Kakoi H, Anniko M, Pettersson CA. Auditory epithelial migration .1. Macroscopic evidence of migration and pathways in rat. Acta Otolaryngol 1996;116(3):435–8.
39. O'Donoghue GM. Epithelial migration on the guinea-pig tympanic membrane: the influence of perforation and ventilating tube insertion. Clin Otolaryngol Allied Sci 1983;8(5):297–303.
40. Miller SM. Epidermal migration in the external ear canal of the guinea pig. J Otolaryngol Soc Aust 1983;5(2):71–5.
41. O'Donoghue GM. Tympanic epithelium: an ultrastructural, experimental and clinical-study. J R Soc Med 1984;77(9):758–60.
42. Johnson A, Hawke M. An ink impregnation study of the migratory skin in the external auditory canal of the guinea-pig. Acta Otolaryngol 1986;101(3–4): 269–77.
43. Tabacca NE, Cole LK, Hillier A, et al. Epithelial migration on the canine tympanic membrane. Vet Dermatol 2011;22(6):502–10.
44. Connors BW. Sensory transduction. In: Boron WF, Boulpaep EL, editors. Medical physiology. updated edition. Philadelphia: Elsevier Saunders; 2005. p. 343–52.
45. Defalque VE, Rosenstein DS, Rosser EJ. Measurement of normal middle ear cavity volume in mesaticephalic dogs. Vet Radiol Ultrasound 2005;46:490–3.
46. Evans HE, de Lahunta A. The respiratory system. In: Evans HE, de Lahunta A, editors. Miller's anatomy of the dog. 4th edition. St. Louis (MO): W. B. Elsevier Saunders; 2013. p. 345.
47. Bluestone CD. Anatomy. Eustachian tube, structure, function, role in otitis media. Hamilton (ON): BC Decker Inc; 2005. 25–50.
48. Cole LK, Samii VF. Contrast-enhanced computed tomographic imaging of the auditory tube in mesaticephalic dogs. Vet Radiol Ultrasound 2007;48:125–8.
49. Michaels L. The ear. In: Sternberg SS, editor. Histology for pathologists. 2nd edition. Philadelphia: Lippincott-Raven; 1997. p. 337–66.
50. Michaels L. Atlas of ear, nose and throat pathology. In: Gresham GA, editor. Current histopathology, vol. 16. Dordrecht (The Netherlands): Kluwer Academic Publishers; 1990. p. 9–39.

Collection and Preparation of Dog and Cat Ears for Histologic Examination

Bradley L. Njaa, DVM, MVSc, DACVP[a],*, Mee Ja M. Sula, DVM[b]

KEYWORDS

- Ear necropsy exam • Otic landmarks • Tissue preparation • Otic decalcification

KEY POINTS

- Instilling fixative solutions into the tympanic bullae immediately following death will ensure excellent tissue preservation of the middle and internal ear.
- Decalcification is the most time-consuming part of tissue processing but is relatively simple, typically reaching the end point in a few weeks.
- Bisecting the ear close to the round window using the landmarks described will allow the pathologist to evaluate all 3 compartments of the ear on a single glass slide.

INTRODUCTION

At the time of necropsy, dog and cat ears have typically been given cursory attention, usually limited to examination of the pinnae and external acoustic meatus (EAM). With the addition of historical or clinical evidence of middle or internal ear disease, tympanic bullae may be opened and examined for gross evidence of exudate or masses; however, a paucity of publications suggest that most cases do not result in histologic evaluation. The complexity of the ear, which includes integument, mucosa, cartilage, bone, and neural tissues, and the special procedures required to allow histologic examination, are 2 of the more common reasons for reluctance by clinicians and pathologists to thoroughly assess the ear.

Most veterinary textbooks provide very little guidance regarding ear sampling, processing, and examination. One of the earliest necropsy procedure texts provides a single sentence suggesting examination of ears along with paranasal sinuses.[1] Even the comprehensive pathology text *Jubb, Kennedy, and Palmer's Pathology of Domestic Animals*, first published in 1963, has provided fewer than 10 pages through

[a] Center for Veterinary Health Sciences, Department of Pathobiology, Oklahoma State University, 226 McElroy Hall, Stillwater, OK 74078-2007, USA; [b] Center for Veterinary Health Sciences, Department of Pathobiology, Oklahoma State University, 250 McElroy Hall, Stillwater, OK 74078-2007, USA
* Corresponding author.
E-mail address: brad.njaa@okstate.edu

Vet Clin Small Anim 42 (2012) 1127–1135
http://dx.doi.org/10.1016/j.cvsm.2012.08.003
0195-5616/12/$ – see front matter © 2012 Elsevier Inc. All rights reserved.

the years on the subject.[2] In the late 1970s, Rose published a series of short articles devoted completely to otology, 2 of which addressed necropsy of the ear.[3,4] A handful of recent publications are beginning to provide more details of otic anatomy, physiology, and pathology in domestic animals.[5–8]

This article is included in this issue to help demystify both the collection and preparation of ear samples, and to briefly describe gross features and key landmarks of the ear. However, it is not the intent to provide an exhaustive account of normal and pathologic findings. For more specific details, the reader is referred to the key articles and texts listed in the references section (specifically Refs.[6–8]).

NECROPSY EXAMINATION AND EAR COLLECTION

Small animal necropsy examination has changed very little over the past 2 centuries. The basic tools necessary include a sharp necropsy knife, tissue forceps, tissue scissors, appropriate tools for cutting through the bone of the ribs, limbs, and calvaria, and containers for tissue collection. In general, a section of most tissues are collected for future histologic examination, further analysis by other ancillary laboratories (ie, parasitology, virology, bacteriology, toxicology, and so forth) or in combination. However, as previously mentioned, portions of the ear are rarely collected or sampled for further analysis. What follows is a stepwise method of collection beginning with removal of the head.

Remove the head from the carcass by opening the atlanto-occipital (A-O) joint ventrally. Gradually open the joint to expose the spinal cord so that it can be cleanly severed from the brainstem. Once the cord is cut, apply gentle traction to the joint such that cutting soft tissues causes the dorsum of the head to flex caudally toward the cervical spine and the A-O joint widens ventrally, disarticulates completely, and allows the head to be freed from the carcass.

At this time, the tympanic bullae should be opened to grossly examine the middle ear cavity. From the ventral aspect, clear the musculature from the ventral surface of the bulla bilaterally (**Fig. 1**). The ventral face of the tympanic bullae should be removed bilaterally to reveal the tympanic cavities (**Fig. 2**). Ideally, sharp, medium-sized Liston bone-cutting forceps[1] should be used. The membrane lining the tympanic cavities should be thin and translucent, and the bony portion of the tympanic bullae should be thin and easily opened. Increases in thickness of either the membrane or bone are most likely indications of previous or ongoing inflammation. Bilateral, even thickening of the tympanic bullae may be present normally in older tomcats. Normal bullae in dogs and cats should be relatively pale with minimal clear fluid within the tympanic cavity. Excess fluid, turbid fluid, suppurative or mucoid exudate, or masses within the tympanic cavity are abnormal. Samples should be collected aseptically to identify and characterize any associated or causative bacterial or viral pathogens.

The tympanic membrane should be examined at this time. Although this can be done without magnification, a much better assessment can be made if an illuminated magnifier or stereomicroscope is used. The normal tympanic membrane is clear to minimally opaque, and held in a slightly taut caudoventrally retracted position by the manubrium of the malleus (**Fig. 3**). Look for evidence of perforations, cloudiness, or thickening of the tympanic membrane. Assess whether the tympanic cavity mucosa is thickened or reddened, both evidence of previous or ongoing otitis media.

---

[1] Many incorrectly refer to these as rongeurs. Bone-cutting forceps have a single, sharp cutting edge whereas rongeurs have concave tips with peripheral cutting edges designed to scoop out pieces of bone.

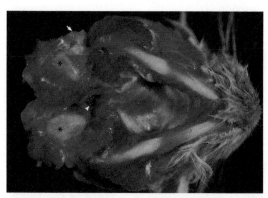

Fig. 1. Ventral view of a cat's head with tympanic bullae (*asterisks*) exposed. Arrow indicates annular cartilage of the right ear, and white arrowhead indicates nasopharyngeal opening. (*Courtesy of* Dr B.L. Njaa, Center for Veterinary Health Sciences, Oklahoma State University, Stillwater, OK.)

Once initial assessment and sampling of the middle ear is complete, sections may be prepared for fixation and further processing. From the dorsal view, make a midline linear incision through the skin that overlies the dorsum of the skull. Reflect each flap of skin lateral to the level of the cartilaginous EAM (horizontal auditory tube). Sever the EAM close to the underlying musculature. After removing the temporal muscles, make a transverse saw cut (cut 1) caudal to the eyes in line with the lateralmost extensions of the zygomatic process of the temporal bone (**Fig. 4**). Then make a saw cut that extends perpendicularly from the first cut caudally to the medial margin of the foramen magnum (cut 2). Repeat this on the contralateral side (cut 3). Carefully remove the calvarium to expose the brain. Occasionally the window created may be too narrow to easily remove the brain. Cuts 2 and 3 can be positioned more laterally; however, be sure these communicate with the medial margins of the foramen magnum caudally to allow for easy removal of the calvarium.

Holding the rostral portion of the skull, gently tap the occipital condyles on a flat surface allowing the rostral portions of the brain to separate from the inner surface of the skull. Using scissors, sever the meningeal attachments as well as the cranial

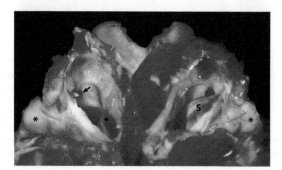

Fig. 2. Opened tympanic bullae in a cat. The opened right tympanic bulla has an intact septum bulla (S). The septum bulla has been opened with the rostral edge left intact (*black arrowhead*) and the round window exposed (*arrow*). Asterisks indicate annular cartilage of the right and left external ears. (*Courtesy of* Dr B.L. Njaa, Center for Veterinary Health Sciences, Oklahoma State University, Stillwater, OK.)

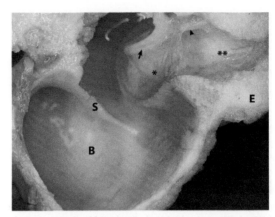

Fig. 3. Rostral view of the right middle and external ear in a dog. The manubrium of the malleus (*arrow*) is embedded in the pars tensa of tympanic membrane (*asterisk*), representing the medial termination of the external acoustic meatus (*double asterisk*). The pars flaccida of the tympanic membrane (*arrowhead*) is partially ruptured, owing to the dissection. B, tympanic bulla; S, incomplete septum bulla; E, ventral bony rim of the external acoustic meatus. (*Courtesy of* Dr B.L. Njaa, Center for Veterinary Health Sciences, Oklahoma State University, Stillwater, OK.)

nerves, freeing the brain from the skull. Moving caudally, once at the level of the petrous portion of the temporal bones, recognized by their distinct pale yellow coloration, carefully sever cranial nerves VII and VIII at the point where they enter the internal acoustic meatus (**Fig. 5**B). This point provides a good opportunity to observe these nerves grossly for any changes such as swelling, discoloration, or exudate.

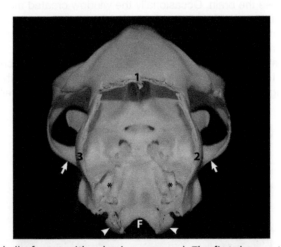

Fig. 4. Opened skull of a cat with calvarium removed. The first dorsorostral saw cut (1) is made caudal to the eyes. A second lateral saw cut connects the first cut through to the medial edge of the ipsilateral occipital condyle (2). The same saw cut is repeated contralaterally (3). Bilaterally, the petrous portions of the temporal bones (*asterisks*) are normally distinctly yellow in fresh tissues but lose this color during maceration. F, foramen magnum; arrowheads indicate occipital condyles, and arrows indicate zygomatic process of the temporal bone. (*Courtesy of* Dr B.L. Njaa, Center for Veterinary Health Sciences, Oklahoma State University, Stillwater, OK.)

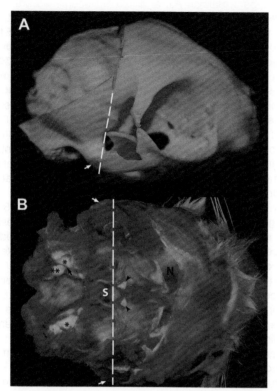

Fig. 5. Landmarks for ear collection in the cat. (*A*) Macerated skull. Once the brain has been removed, extend the first rostral saw cut (*dashed line*) through the floor of the skull and through the lateralmost edge of the zygomatic process of the temporal bone (*arrow*). (*B*) Fresh skull. Extend the saw cut through the floor of the skull (*dashed line*) through the sella turcica (S) caudal to the optic nerves (*black arrowheads*) and through the lateralmost edge of the zygomatic process of the temporal bone (*white arrows*). Cranial nerves VII and VIII (*double asterisk*) exit the skull through the internal acoustic meatus (*black arrow*) of the petrous portion of the temporal bone (*asterisk*). N, frontal sinus. (*A and B Courtesy of* Dr B.L. Njaa, Center for Veterinary Health Sciences, Oklahoma State University, Stillwater, OK.)

Continue severing the remainder of the cranial nerves and meninges caudally, releasing the brainstem and cerebellum.

With the brain removed, extend your original cut (cut 1) ventrally through the base of the skull (**Fig. 5**A). This action will cut through the zygomatic process of the temporal bones bilaterally at their most lateral extensions (original landmarks for cut 1). Once the bones are severed through the floor of the skull (see **Fig. 5**B) the prosector should have the skull severed in 2, with the caudal portion containing integral portions for complete ear examination. At this point the caudal portion of the skull may be placed in 10% buffered formalin for tissue fixation. Additional trimming of remaining temporal bone is optional, but may decrease the required fixation and decalcification period. Ensure that both bullae are opened to maximize tissue penetration by the fixative.[9,10]

TISSUE PREPARATION

Immersion fixation in 10% formalin followed by tissue embedding in paraffin is the most common method of tissue preparation for routine samples in veterinary medicine. This technique is very efficient, rapid, and effective for most tissues, but requires that the tissues be soft enough to cut with thin microtome blades. Tissues that have a high concentration of calcium, such as bone or teeth, are not soft enough for paraffin embedding. Microtome sectioning through hard tissues results in various artifacts that can render the tissue sections impossible to evaluate while destroying microtome blades. Therefore, to use paraffin-embedding techniques for hard, calcified structures, the tissues must be softened through a process that removes calcium and is aptly termed decalcification.

The first critical step of preparation of tissues that contain bone is thorough fixation. Several commercial decalcifying products also contain a fixative, but if they do not, tissues must be immersed in 10% buffered formalin for a minimum of 48 hours with a minimum ratio of 10 parts formalin to 1 part tissue. Following complete fixation, the decalcification process can be initiated.[11]

For most bony structures, saws may be used to create thin slab sections so that tissue-processing times can be minimized. The bony compartments of the middle and internal ear are intricately connected but differ greatly, rending a saw far too destructive for sectioning. The bone of tympanic bullae and EAMs is cancellous, comprising a mixture of bony trabeculae and marrow compartments. The septum bulla is very thin cancellous bone that typically lacks the marrow cavities but is made up of trabecular bone.[8]

The petrous portion of the temporal bone is extremely dense and forms the dorsomedial margin of the tympanic cavity. It is a roughly triangular wedge of bone that is typically a deeper yellow than surrounding squamous temporal bone. The growth pattern of this bone is neither lamellated nor woven, but rather a mixture. It lacks marrow compartments and instead is a mixture of calcified cartilaginous matrix (also known as globuli ossei) interwoven with primitive bone that replaces lacunar spaces created by degenerated chondrocytes.[12] Ironically, this bone tends to decalcify more thoroughly and quickly than the cancellous bony portions of the temporal and occipital bones.

Buried deep within this dense bone is the delicate membranous labyrinth of the vestibular system and cochlea. These fluid-filled compartments contain thin, flexible membranes and delicate, terminally divided, nonrenewable sensory hair cells. The process of decalcification and softening of bone must be sufficient to allow paraffin embedding while at the same time resulting in minimal artifactual damage to these sensory tissues.

The decalcification process is a chemical reaction that involves acid decalcification, calcium chelation, or a combination of these 2 methods. Most veterinary diagnostic histology laboratories use commercial products that contain various percentages of acids, typically formic acid, along with buffers and possibly fixative. One product used by many laboratories is Leica Decalcifier 1, which incorporates 12% formic acid, 6% formaldehyde, and 2% methanol.[13] The decalcification process depends on repeated and regular replacement of the decalcifier solution and the size of the ear being processed. Using the Leica Decalcifier 1 a cat ear takes approximately 7 to 14 days for proper end-point decalcification, whereas ears from a medium-sized dog may take 2 to 3 weeks.

Recently, Lafond and colleagues[14] compared 4 different solutions to evaluate their ability to decalcify canine ears. The solutions included: (1) 22% formic acid; (2) 5% formic acid; (3) PFF[2], composed of aqueous saturated picric acid, 37% to 40%

---

[2] PFF may be of limited utility in diagnostic laboratories owing to the necessity of constant refrigeration conditions and inherent dangers associated with storing picric acid.

formaldehyde, and 88% to 90% formic acid; and (4) ethylenediamine tetra-acetic acid (EDTA, a chelator). Formic acid at 22% rapidly decalcified the tissue in less than 2 weeks but resulted in severe artifacts. PFF slowed the decalcification times (5–6 weeks) but resulted in fewer artifacts. EDTA resulted in the best preservation with fewest artifacts, but took over 3 months to reach the end point.

ANATOMIC LANDMARKS FOR TISSUE SECTIONING

The ideal method for assessing the 3 compartments of the ear is to perform serial step sections through the entire block of tissue, resulting in a few hundred slides per ear.[10] This method is extremely expensive and cost prohibitive for most veterinary diagnostic pathology laboratories, and would further prevent pathologists and laboratories from exploring otic pathology.

An alternative method is to cut through the ear in a manner that will allow visualization and examination of a majority of all 3 compartments. Although this is performed on tissues that have undergone extensive decalcification, the landmarks are depicted in tissue from a cat that have not yet undergone decalcification (**Fig. 6**). Because bullae will have been opened to ensure proper fixation, this allows visualization of the important landmarks. Microtome blades, if available, are ideal because they are particularly sharp and thin, resulting in minimal displacement of fine structures while trimming. Razor blades are also effective, although slightly more bulky when dealing with fine anatomic structures. Orientate a sharp new blade in the middle third of the occipital condyle, about 1 to 2 mm medial to the round window midway through where the auricular cartilage apposes the bony opening of the EAM. The result is a section of ear that includes the tympanic bulla and bone, vestibule and cochlea of the inner ear, and an often narrow section through the EAM that includes tympanic membrane and manubrium of the malleus (**Fig. 7**). Thus, nearly all portions of the ear can be histologically examined. However, there is a greater tendency for delicate membranes of the inner ear to be broken or displaced, introducing greater artifact to the membranous labyrinth.

In cases with clinical signs of inner ear disease, the entire ear can be embedded and step-sectioned as is routinely performed in human otic pathology. Alternatively, the petrous portion of the temporal bone can be carefully dissected from the ear and

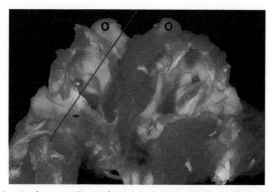

Fig. 6. Ear sectioning in the cat. Align a fresh blade through the middle third of the occipital condyle (O), a few millimeters medial to the round window, and through the external acoustic meatus a few millimeters lateral to the medial extremity of the annular cartilage of the ear (*arrow*). (*Courtesy of* Dr M.M. Sula, Center for Veterinary Health Sciences, Oklahoma State University, Stillwater, OK.)

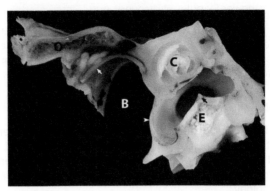

Fig. 7. Decalcified section of ear in a cat. Portions of all 3 ear compartments are present in this section, including the cochlea (C) of the inner ear, the tympanic cavity (B) bound by the bone of the tympanic bulla (*white arrow*), and the external ear (E), within which is an abundance of keratin and debris. The tympanic membrane is too thin to easily visualize, but the manubrium of the malleus (*black arrow*) is embedded in this membrane. The occipital bone (O) is cancellous bone with a marrow compartment. White arrowhead indicates septum bulla. (*Courtesy of* Dr M.M. Sula, Center for Veterinary Health Sciences, Oklahoma State University, Stillwater, OK.)

directly placed in fixative. Once decalcified, the entire bony and membranous labyrinth can be sectioned to ensure that the semicircular canals of the vestibular system, as well as the vestibule and cochlea and associated ganglia and cranial nerves, are thoroughly examined.

The decalcification process using formic acid is harsh to nucleic acids. When these tissues are placed on slides for routine staining, they tend to be pale and more eosinophilic than normal with less hematoxylin-stained, basophilic contrast. To help alleviate this problem of pallor, tissues should be thoroughly rinsed before embedding and the histology laboratory informed that slides need prolonged staining with hematoxylin. Approximately twice the usual length of hematoxylin staining works well.

SUMMARY

Although external otic disease has been well characterized in veterinary medicine by dermatologists and dermatopathologists, the middle and internal ear compartments have been largely neglected for decades. Despite its complexity, it is hoped that the simple procedures outlined and described in this article for ear removal, processing, and examination will encourage more practitioners and pathologists to delve into the fascinating world of otology and otic pathology.

REFERENCES

1. Jones TC, Gleiser CA. Veterinary necropsy procedures. Philadelphia: J.B. Lippincott Co; 1954. p. 43–62.
2. Jubb KV, Kennedy PC. 1st edition. Pathology of domestic animals, vol. 2. New York: Academic Press; 1963. p. 475–83.
3. Rose WR. Necropsy of the ear—1: gross examination. Vet Med Small Anim Clin 1978;73:637–9.
4. Rose WR. Necropsy—2: pathology of middle ear and biopsy. Vet Med Small Anim Clin 1978;73:764–7.

5. Heine PA. Anatomy of the ear. Vet Clin North Am Small Animal Pract 2004;34: 379–95.
6. Cole LK. Anatomy and physiology of the canine ear. Vet Dermatol 2009;20: 412–21.
7. König HE, Liebich HG. Veterinary anatomy of domestic mammals: textbook and colour atlas. 3rd edition. New York: Schattauer; 2007. p. 593–608.
8. Njaa BL, Wilcock BP. The ear and eye. In: Pathologic basis of veterinary disease. 5th edition. Elsevier; 2011. p. 1153–93.
9. Schuknecht HF. Pathology of the ear. Cambridge (United Kingdom): Harvard University Press; 1974. p. 3–20.
10. Merchant SN, Nadol JB. Schuknecht's pathology of the ear. 3rd edition. Shelton (CT): People's Medical Publishing House; 2010. p. 13–95.
11. Carson FL. Histotechnology: a self-instructional text. Chicago: ASCP Press; 1997. p. 38–40.
12. Michaels L. The ear. In: Histology for pathologists. 2nd edition. New York: Lippincott-Raven; 2007. p. 337–66.
13. MSDS No. 130Decalcifier 1. Richmond (IL): Leica Biosystems Richmond, Inc; 2011.
14. Lafond JF, Henning G, Lejeune T, et al. Processing of canine and non-human primate inner ear for histopathological evaluation. In: Proceedings of the 31st annual Society for Toxicologic Pathology symposium, Boston; June 24–27, 2012. Montreal (Canada): Charles River.

Primary Secretory Otitis Media in Cavalier King Charles Spaniels

Lynette K. Cole, DVM, MS, DACVD

KEYWORDS

- Primary secretory otitis media • PSOM • Otitis media with effusion • OME
- Cavalier King Charles spaniel • Myringotomy

KEY POINTS

- Signs suggestive of primary secretory otitis media include hearing loss, neck scratching, otic pruritus, head shaking, abnormal yawning, head tilt, facial paralysis, or vestibular disturbances, with an individual Cavalier King Charles spaniel presenting with one or multiple signs.
- A large, bulging pars flaccida identified on otoscopic examination confirms the diagnosis.
- In many Cavalier King Charles spaniels with primary secretory otitis media the pars flaccida is flat, and radiographic imaging (eg, computed tomography, magnetic resonance imaging) is needed to confirm the diagnosis.
- Current treatment of primary secretory otitis media includes performing a myringotomy into the caudal-ventral quadrant of the pars tensa with subsequent flushing of the mucus out of the bulla using a video otoscope.
- Until a treatment is found to prevent the mucus from recurring or the cause of the disease is identified and controlled, repeat myringotomies and flushing of the middle ear will be needed to keep the middle ear free of mucus.

INTRODUCTION

Primary secretory otitis media (PSOM) is a disease that has been described in the Cavalier King Charles spaniel (CKCS) in a retrospective study by Stern-Bertholtz and colleagues[1] reporting on 61 cases of PSOM in 43 CKCS. CKCS diagnosed with PSOM in this report exhibited head and neck pain, spontaneous vocalization, and a guarded and horizontal neck carriage (64%); neurologic signs (ataxia, facial paralysis, nystagmus, head tilt or seizures) (25%), otic pruritus without otitis externa (15%), otitis externa (15%), impaired hearing (13%), and fatigue (7%), with 46% having a combination of signs. The male to female ratio was 23:20, and the age at presentation was between 2 and 10 years of age, with 86% between 3 and 7 years old. Some

The author has nothing to disclose.
Department of Veterinary Clinical Sciences, College of Veterinary Medicine, The Ohio State University, 601 Vernon Tharp Street, Columbus, OH 43210, USA
E-mail address: cole.143@osu.edu

dogs were suspected to have cervical disease before PSOM was recognized as a clinical entity, and radiographic examination of the cervical spine was performed in 17 dogs and myelography performed in 5 dogs. The diagnosis in 57 of 61 episodes of PSOM was made based on visualization of a bulging, opaque, but intact tympanic membrane with an operating microscope, and the finding of an accumulation of mucus in the middle ear after myringotomy, whereas in 4 of 61 episodes the tympanic membrane was already ruptured and the mucus plug was visualized. The highly viscous, opaque, grayish or yellowish solid plug appeared to fill the entire middle ear, and was either removed in one piece with micro ear forceps or by flushing it loose and lifting it out with the tip of a suction catheter.[1] No additional tests were used to evaluate the dogs for PSOM, so early disease may have been missed. In addition, the actual anatomic region of the tympanic membrane that was bulging (ie, pars flaccida, pars tensa) was not described in this study.

CLINICAL SIGNS OF PSOM

In some CKCS with PSOM, clinical signs may be subtle.[2] In two studies where magnetic resonance imaging (MRI) was performed on clinically normal CKCS (one pre-breeding syringomyelia screening test[3] and one screening for Chiari-like malformation and syringomyelia[4]), material hyperintense to cerebral gray matter on T2-weighted images was identified in the bulla in 10 of 23 CKCS (43%; 6 of 10 [60%] bilateral, 4 of 10 [40%] unilateral)[3] and 37 of 68 CKCS (54%; 17 of 37 [46%] bilateral, 20 of 37 [54%] unilateral).[4] In the study by Harcourt-Brown and colleagues,[3] there was no significant difference in the mean ages of those with material (30 months) and without material (34 months) in the bulla; however, the youngest dog with material in the bulla was 25 months, in contrast to the youngest dog without material in the bulla being only 10 months old. Another study evaluating neurologic signs and MRI results in CKCS with the Chiari-like malformation identified 11 of 40 (28%) CKCS to have material in the bulla (4 of 11 [36%] bilateral, 7 of 11 [64%] unilateral), and none of these dogs showed any clinical or neurologic sign of middle ear disease; however, all had clinical signs affecting the brain and/or cranial nerves (cranial group) or spine (spinal group).[5]

POST-MYRINGOTOMY TREATMENT AND FOLLOW-UP OF PSOM

In the Stern-Bertholtz and colleagues[1] retrospective study, treatment postmyringotomy for PSOM consisted of multiple combinations of topical and systemic medications. All dogs were treated corticosteroids consisting of topical betamethasone (85%) and/or systemic prednisolone (82%). Additional systemic treatments consisted of antibiotics (92%) and/or a mucolytic (57%) (acetylcysteine or bromhexine) while 10% received a topical antibiotic solution. The dogs were reexamined under anesthesia within 7 to 20 days after the first visit, and had all improved or were asymptomatic per the owner's assessment; however, the middle ears again contained mucus and were reflushed. The mucus at the follow-up visit was noted to be less viscous and solid than it had been on initial presentation. Healing of the tympanic membrane was noted in the record of 42 CKCS, with 25% of the tympanic membranes healing within 7 days postmyringotomy and 69% healing after 8 or more days. Of the 51 cases for which the owners pursued treatment, 14 required 2 revisits, 10 required 4 revisits, 2 required 5 revisits, and 4 required 6 revisits for reflushing of the middle ear before the middle ear was found to be clear of mucus. Twelve dogs had 1 or more relapses of PSOM after 6 to 18 months.[1] At present, the cause of PSOM is unknown; however, it has been speculated to be due to a dysfunction of the middle ear or auditory tube (increased production of mucus in the middle ear) or decreased drainage of the middle ear through the auditory tube, or both. Until a treatment is found to prevent the mucus from recurring or the cause of the disease is identified and controlled, the fact that these CKCS had a relapse of PSOM is not surprising.

POSSIBLE PATHOGENESIS OF PSOM

Dysfunction of the auditory tube is implicated in the pathogenesis of otitis media with effusion (OME) in humans, which may be similar to PSOM in CKCS, and in humans may occur secondary to craniofacial abnormalities such as cleft palate. Hayes and colleagues[4] evaluated the relationship between nasopharyngeal conformation and OME in CKCS (the test brachycephalic group) in comparison with boxers (the brachycephalic control group) and cocker spaniels (the mesocephalic control group). Two objective measures of nasopharyngeal conformation were evaluated: the thickness of the soft palate on a midline sagittal MRI and the cross-sectional area (dorsoventral height and width) of the nasopharynx at the level of the rostral border of the tympanic bulla on a transverse view. Dogs with a signal void on MRI in the bulla were considered unaffected, whereas dogs with material hyperintense to cerebral gray matter in one or both bullae on T2-weighted images were considered to have unilateral or bilateral OME, respectively.[4]

There was a significant difference in the incidence of OME in the brachycephalic group (CKCS and boxers combined) compared with the mesocephalic group (cocker spaniels—none had OME); however, there was no significant difference between the incidence of OME in the CKCS and boxers ($P = .07$). When looking at the CKCS group only, there was a significant difference in the thickness of the soft palate and the cross-sectional area of the nasopharynx between those CKCS with bilateral OME and those without OME; however, no significant differences were found between those CKCS with unilateral OME and those with bilateral OME or no OME. No significant differences were found in the thickness of the soft palate and the cross-sectional area of the nasopharynx for the boxers, irrespective of whether they had unilateral OME, bilateral OME, or no OME. Based on the results of this study, there was an association between OME and the brachycephalic conformation; furthermore, specifically for the CKCS breed, those with bilateral OME had a significantly greater thickness of the soft palate and reduced cross-sectional area of the nasopharynx compared with CKCS without OME. The study demonstrates an association between changes in the nasopharyngeal soft tissues and the incidence of OME, but cannot predict the nature of this relationship.[4] These anatomic changes in the nasopharynx may impair auditory tube drainage.

BREED PREDILECTION AND PSOM

PSOM appears to be overrepresented in the CKCS breed. In dogs diagnosed with the Chiari-like malformation by MRI and computed tomography (CT), 38.7% had concurrent PSOM with the prevalence being significantly greater in the CKCS than in the non-CKCS.[6] In addition to the CKCS, other breeds may have PSOM. Stern-Bertholtz and colleagues[1] report identifying PSOM in a boxer, a dachshund, and a shih tzu, and the control brachycephalic breed in the study by Hayes and colleagues[4] was a group of 28 boxers, of which 9 (32%) had OME.

TYMPANOSTOMY TUBES AND PSOM

Tympanostomy tubes have been used in human medicine to provide continual tympanic cavity ventilation and pressure equalization for the treatment of OME. Two studies have been published using tympanostomy tubes as an alternative treatment to myringotomy and middle ear flushes in CKCS with OME/PSOM.[7,8] In both studies the insertion of the tympanostomy tube provided relief of the presenting clinical signs for a maximum of 8 months. The CKCS in the first study[7] had unilateral OME that was first treated surgically with a lateral wall resection, before the insertion of the tympanostomy tube. Lumen occlusion of the tympanostomy tube with wax and hair occurred 5 weeks after tympanostomy insertion, which was resolved using microcrocodile forceps to remove the exudate. Recurrence of clinical signs returned after 8 months. On examination, the tympanostomy tube had been extruded and the tympanic membrane had healed, so another myringotomy was performed, revealing a recurrence of the middle ear effusion. The effusion was aspirated and a new tympanostomy tube was inserted.[7] In a second study,[8] 3 CKCS had tympanostomy tubes inserted as treatment for PSOM. In all 3 cases, at least one myringotomy had been performed before the insertion of the tympanostomy tubes. Initial improvement postmyringotomy was noted in all dogs; however, clinical signs returned within 2 to 4 weeks. After insertion of the tympanostomy tube, the CKCS were symptom-free for 8, 6, and 3 months as noted either on examination (1 CKCS) or as reported by the owner (2 CKCS).[8] Insertion of a tympanostomy tube may be an alternative to repeated myringotomy and middle ear flushes for the treatment of PSOM, but requires specialized equipment (eg, operating microscope) as well as training to perform the procedure.

HEARING LOSS AND PSOM

In children, OME can cause impaired language and speech development because of hearing loss, which may lead to learning disabilities. PSOM can lead to hearing loss in the CKCS. Hearing assessment in the dog is performed using electrodiagnostic testing. The brain responds to sensory stimuli by changes in electrical activity. These changes can be recorded and are referred to as evoked responses. Brainstem auditory-evoked responses (BAER) can be used in the dog to help characterize hearing loss. The BAER is a far-field recording of neuroelectrical activity of the auditory nerve and brainstem pathways in response to a sound stimulus (electrodiagnostic evaluation of auditory function in the dog is discussed in the article by Scheifele and colleagues elsewhere in this issue). Hearing loss is categorized as either sensorineural or conductive in origin. Sensorineural hearing loss may be due to injury to the cochlear hair cells in the inner ear (sensory) or to the auditory nerve (neural). Conductive hearing loss is due to abnormal propagation of sound through the external, middle, and inner ears.[9]

In a study by Harcourt-Brown and colleagues[3] the investigators evaluated the effect of the middle ear effusions in CKCS with PSOM on the BAER. In this study using BAER testing with subsequent analysis of the latency-intensity function, the middle ear effusion in the CKCS was associated with a mean conductive hearing loss of 21 dB relative to normal hearing level (dB nHL). Middle ear effusion was associated with an elevated BAER threshold; however, there was variability between individual cavaliers. Some cavaliers with a middle ear effusion had a normal BAER threshold (<30 dB nHL), whereas in others the BAER threshold was markedly elevated (eg, 100 dB nHL).[3] None of the owners reported any hearing loss in their CKCS in this study[3] whereas in the study by Stern-Bertholtz and colleagues,[1] impaired hearing was reported as a presenting sign of PSOM in 13% of the cases.

DIAGNOSIS OF PSOM

Signs suggestive of PSOM include hearing loss, neck scratching, otic pruritus, head shaking, abnormal yawning, head tilt, facial paralysis, or vestibular disturbances, with an individual CKCS presenting with one or multiple signs. However, none of these clinical signs may be considered pathognomonic for PSOM. Evaluation of a CKCS with suspected PSOM should begin with an otic examination. If a large, bulging pars flaccida is identified (**Fig. 1**), the diagnosis is made, and no other tests are required.[10] However, in many CKCS with PSOM the pars flaccida is flat,[3,10] and radiographic imaging (eg, CT, MRI) is needed to confirm the diagnosis.

MANAGEMENT OF PSOM

Although there are 2 reports in the veterinary literature regarding the use of tympanostomy tubes for treatment of PSOM,[7,8] no long-term prospective studies have been published on the outcome after extrusion of the tympanostomy tubes as far as the length of time the bulla remains effusion free. In addition, no studies have reported on the efficacy of a more "permanent" or long-term tympanostomy tube for treatment of PSOM. The treatment commonly used at present involves performing a myringotomy into the caudal-ventral quadrant of the pars tensa with subsequent flushing of the mucus from the bulla with the aid of a video otoscope or operating microscope. In CKCS with hearing loss, pre- and postflush air- and bone-conducted BAER testing is recommended to determine the extent of the hearing loss and whether the hearing loss is conductive owing to the accumulation of mucus in the middle ear, or if the hearing loss is sensorineural and is unrelated to the PSOM.

Postflushing medications dispensed may include a short course of prednisone (0.5–1 mg/kg every 24 hours for 7 days, then taper to every other day for 2–3 weeks) for the swelling and inflammation that may occur after flushing, and a broad-spectrum systemic antibiotic to help prevent a postflushing bacterial otitis externa. Unfortunately, because the primary cause of this disease is not known, the mucus may recur.[1,7,8] Reported treatments that did not appear to prevent the recurrence of the mucus include topical otic glucocorticoids,[1] systemic glucocorticoids,[1,7] systemic antibiotics,[1] topical otic antibiotics,[1] and mucolytic agents[1]; however, use of the

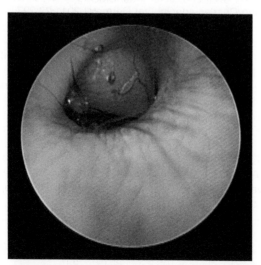

Fig. 1. Video otoscopic image of a bulging pars flaccida in a Cavalier King Charles spaniel with primary secretory otitis media (PSOM). (*Courtesy of* Dr Cole, The Ohio State University, Columbus, OH; with permission.)

over-the-counter timed-release mucolytic *N*-acetylcysteine (600 mg every 24 hours) may help to extend the symptom-free time, although no prospective studies have been performed to determine the efficacy of this treatment in the management of PSOM.

REFERENCES

1. Stern-Bertholtz W, Sjostrom L, Wallin Hakanson N. Primary secretory otitis media in the Cavalier King Charles spaniel: a review of 61 cases. J Small Anim Pract 2003;44:253–6.
2. Volk HA. Middle ear effusions in dogs: an incidental finding? Vet J 2011;188: 256–7.
3. Harcourt-Brown TR, Parker JE, Granger N, et al. Effect of middle ear effusion on the brain-stem auditory evoked response of Cavalier King Charles spaniels. Vet J 2011;188:341–5.
4. Hayes GM, Friend EJ, Jeffrey ND. Relationship between pharyngeal conformation and otitis media with effusion in CKCS. Vet Rec 2010;167:55–8.
5. Lu D, Lamb CR, Pfeiffer DU, et al. Neurological signs and results of magnetic resonance imaging in 40 cavalier King Charles spaniels with Chiari type 1-like malformations. Vet Rec 2003;153:260–3.
6. Loughlin CA, Marino DJ, Govier S. Primary secretory otitis media (PSOM) in dogs with suspected Chiari-like malformation: 120 cases (2007-2010). Vet Dermatol 2011;22:297.
7. Cox CL, Slack RW, Cox GJ. Insertion of a transtympanic ventilation tube for the treatment of otitis media with effusion. J Small Anim Pract 1989;30:517–9.
8. Corfield GS, Burrows AK, Imani P, et al. The method of application and short term results of tympanostomy tubes for the treatment of primary secretory otitis media in three CKCS dogs. Aust Vet J 2008;86:88–94.
9. Wilson WJ, Mills PC. Brainstem auditory-evoked response in dogs. Am J Vet Res 2005;66:2177–87.
10. Cole LK, Samii VF, Wagner S, et al. Diagnosis of primary secretory otitis media in the cavalier King Charles spaniel. Vet Dermatol 2011;22:297.

Neurological Manifestations of Ear Disease in Dogs and Cats

Laurent S. Garosi, DVM, MRCVS[a],*,
Mark L. Lowrie, MA, VetMB, MVM, MRCVS[a],
Natalie F. Swinbourne, BVM&S, MRCVS[b]

KEYWORDS

* Ear • Vestibular • Horner syndrome • Facial nerve • Deafness

KEY POINTS

* Facial paralysis is the most common neurologic complication following total ear canal ablation lateral bulla osteotomy in dogs and cats.
* Corneal health is the most important management concern with facial nerve paralysis.
* Otitis media and/or interna are the most common cause of vestibular syndrome in dogs and cats.
* Horner syndrome is often seen as a complication of surgery for middle ear disease and especially ventral bulla osteotomy in cats.

INTRODUCTION

The ear serves as the organ of hearing and balance in vertebrates.[1,2] Because of the neuroanatomical structures associated with the different ear structures (facial nerve, sympathetic supply to the eye, vestibular receptor organ, cochlea, and vestibulocochlear nerve), ear diseases can be associated with an array of neurologic manifestations. Facial nerve paralysis and/or Horner syndrome (HS) may occur on the same side as middle ear disease, whereas the clinical signs of inner ear disease in the dog and cat are usually those of a peripheral vestibular syndrome (**Boxes 1** and **2**).[3] Although deafness may also be caused by inner ear disease, it may not be clinically evident with unilateral involvement.

NEUROANATOMICAL STRUCTURES ASSOCIATED WITH THE EAR

Four neuroanatomical structures are associated with the ear: facial nerve, ocular sympathetic tract, vestibular receptors, and cochlea. A good knowledge of the

[a] Davies Veterinary Specialists, Manor Farm Business Park, Higham Gobion SG5 3HR, UK;
[b] Department of Veterinary Clinical Sciences, Royal Veterinary College, Hatfield, UK
* Corresponding author.
E-mail address: lsg@vetspecialists.co.uk

Vet Clin Small Anim 42 (2012) 1143–1160
http://dx.doi.org/10.1016/j.cvsm.2012.08.006
0195-5616/12/$ – see front matter © 2012 Elsevier Inc. All rights reserved.

Box 1
Signs and causes of facial nerve paralysis

Signs

Ipsilateral drooping of ear and lip

Widened palpebral fissure

Drooling

Absence of spontaneous and provoked blinking

Absence of nostril abduction during inspiration

Deviation of nostril toward normal side (unless chronic case in which nostril deviated to affected side and lips retracted farther than normal)

Neurogenic keratoconjunctivitis and dry nose (involvement of parasympathetic supply of lacrimal and nasal glands respectively)

Facial spasms

Causes

Otitis media

Middle ear masses (neoplasia, polyps)

Head and/or peripheral nerve trauma

Intracranial neoplasia

Hypothyroidism

Potentiated sulfonamides

Polyneuropathies

Iatrogenic—complications of total ear canal ablation lateral bulla osteotomy

Idiopathic (most common)

---

neuroanatomy and function of these structures is essential in understanding how ear disease can be associated with neurologic signs.

Facial Nerve

The facial nerve or cranial nerve (CN) VII is a mixed nerve providing somatic and visceral innervation. It provides motor innervation to the muscles of facial expression and the caudal portion of the digastricus muscle (general somatic efferent [GSE] function), and sensory innervation (providing the sense of taste) to the rostral two-thirds of the tongue and palate (parasympathetic general visceral afferent function).[4] In addition, the parasympathetic general visceral efferent component of the facial nerve innervates the lacrimal glands, the glands of the nasal mucosa, and the mandibular and sublingual salivary glands. Finally, the facial nerve has a small contingent of general somatic afferent fibers that supply the concave surface of the auricle of the ear.[5] The somatic efferent fibers in the facial nerve have their cell body located in the facial nucleus in the rostral medulla oblongata. The axons pass through the internal acoustic meatus of the petrosal bone on the dorsal surface of the vestibulocochlear nerve and travel within the facial canal that ultimately emerges at the stylomastoid foramen. As it travels through the temporal bone, the facial canal opens into the cavity of the middle ear lateral to the vestibular window (**Fig. 1**), leaving the facial nerve briefly exposed to the middle ear cavity.[6] After leaving the skull through the stylomastoid

Box 2
Signs and causes of peripheral and central vestibular syndrome

Signs

Unilateral

   Head tilt

   Ataxia

   Falling, leaning, rolling

   Circling

   Nystagmus (spontaneous or positional)

   Strabismus—positional

Bilateral

   Head swaying from side to side

   Head tilt is not observed

   Loss of balance on either side

   Symmetric ataxia with crouched posture

   Inability to elicit physiologic nystagmus

Causes of peripheral vestibular disease

Otogenic infections (otitis media and/or interna)

Nasopharyngeal polyps

Head trauma

Aminoglycosides, topical iodophors, or chlorhexidine

Congenital vestibular disease

Hypothyroidism

Acute idiopathic peripheral vestibular disease

Middle and/or inner ear tumor

Causes of central vestibular disease

Brain infarct or hemorrhage

Infectious encephalitis (distemper, *Toxoplasma*, *Neospora*, fungal, bacterial, rickettsial, feline infectious peritonitis, Cryptococcus)

Meningoencephalitis of unknown cause (granulomatous meningoencephalitis, idiopathic)

Head trauma

Metronidazole toxicity

Intracranial intra-arachnoid cyst

Dermoid and/or epidermoid cyst

Dandy-Walker syndrome

Chiari-like malformation

Hydrocephalus

Primary and/or metastatic brain tumor

Thiamine deficiency

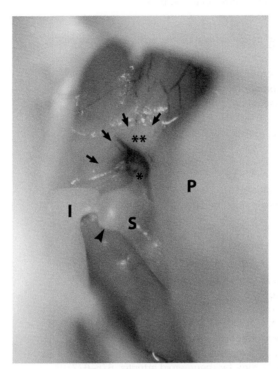

Fig. 1. Caudoventral view of the right middle ear of a cat. The facial nerve (*double asterisk*) passes through the internal acoustic meatus of the petrous portion of the temporal bone. It then courses through the facial canal before exiting caudal to the external acoustic meatus. A small region of the facial canal lacks a complete bony covering (*arrows* follow the rim of the bone of the facial canal). In these regions, the tendon of the stapedius muscle emerges and attaches to the head of the stapes (*asterisks*). Long crus of the incus (I), stapes (S), and promontory of the petrous portion of the temporal bone (P), incudostapedial joint (*arrowhead*). (*Courtesy of* Dr B.L. Njaa, Center for Veterinary Health Sciences, Oklahoma State University, Columbus, OH.)

foramen caudal to the external acoustic meatus, the branches of the facial nerves are distributed to the muscles of facial expression (ear, eyelids, nose, cheeks, lips) and to the caudal portion of the digastric muscle.[7] The parasympathetic division of the facial nerve also has components located near the ear. The parasympathetic nucleus of the facial nerve is located caudal to the genu of the facial nerve (axons from the facial nucleus forming a loop around the abducent nucleus). These fibers join the facial GSE neurons and enter the internal acoustic meatus. Whereas the GSE neurons emerge from the stylomastoid foramen, the general visceral efferent neurons branch off the facial nerve in the major petrosal nerve and chorda tympani nerves.[7] The major petrosal nerve emerges through a small foramen in the pterygoid muscles. It supplies innervation to the lacrimal glands and nasal mucosa. After traveling in the petrous temporal bone, the chorda tympani nerve travels freely through the middle ear before branching off to carry fibers to the taste buds and salivary glands.

Ocular Sympathetic Tract

The ocular sympathetic tract is a three-neuron pathway with the third neuron passing through the tympanic cavity. The cell bodies of the first order neuron (or upper motor neuron) are situated in the hypothalamus and rostral midbrain. These fibers descend the cervical spinal cord in the lateral tectotegmentospinal tract to reach T1 to T3.[8] The first order neurons then synapse on the cell bodies of the lower motor neuron, which is divided into the preganglionic (second order) and postganglionic (third order) neurons. The preganglionic axons leave the vertebral canal via the spinal nerve in the segmental ramus communicans, which joins the thoracic sympathetic trunk. The thoracic sympathetic trunk courses inside the thorax ventrolaterally to the vertebral column and continues cranially as the cervical sympathetic trunk and vagosympathetic trunk within the carotid sheath. The fibers then synapse with the bodies of the postganglionic cells in the cranial cervical ganglion, which lies deep to the tympanic bulla.[8] Some of the postganglionic axons pass through the tympanic bulla, whereas others run medial to it before entering the middle cranial fossa to join the ophthalmic branch of the trigeminal nerve running to the orbit.[9] The sympathetic nervous system innervates and provides tone to the smooth muscle in the periorbita and the eyelids. This tone keeps the globe protruded and the eyelids and third eyelid retracted, causing the palpebral fissure to widen and the third eyelid to be pulled ventrally. The tone of the iris dilator muscle is also maintained by the sympathetic system, which keeps the pupil partially dilated in normal conditions and dilates it during periods of darkness, stress, fear, and painful stimuli.[10]

Vestibular Receptor

The inner ear structures are made up of the bony and membranous labyrinths housed within the petrous portion of the temporal bone. The bony labyrinth is divided into three main contiguous regions: the semicircular canals, the vestibule, and the cochlea. The lumen of each of these structures is filled with perilymph. Two important sensory receptor organs are housed within the bony labyrinths of the inner ear: the vestibular receptor and cochlea.

The vestibular system consists of special proprioceptors within the petrous temporal bone, the vestibular nerve, and four brainstem nuclei located in the rostral medulla oblongata on each side of the fourth ventricle. Its main function is to control balance and it usually prevents the animal from falling over by maintaining and adapting the position of the eyes, head, and body with respect to gravity. The vestibular portion of the membranous labyrinth consists of two major sets of endolymph-filled special proprioceptors: (1) three semicircular ducts, located at approximately right angles to each other and (2) a pair of saclike structures called the utricle and saccule.[11] The semicircular ducts are contained within the semicircular canals whereas the saccule and utricle are within the vestibule. Each semicircular duct has an enlargement at one end, called the ampulla, which contains a hair cell receptor organ called the crista ampullaris. The maculae are the receptors located in the membranous utriculus and saccule. The macula of the saccule is oriented in a vertical plane whereas the macula of the utriculus is in a horizontal plane.[11] These hair cell receptor organs detect the position and movement of the head in space while the animal is standing at rest or when it is moving. The semicircular ducts detect rotatory acceleration and deceleration of the head, whereas the saccule and utricle detect linear acceleration and deceleration and static tilt of the head in space. The information on the position of the head is converted by the hair cells into electrical signals that are sent via the vestibular nerve to the brain. The superior division of the vestibular nerve innervates the macula of the utricle and crista of the anterior and lateral semicircular duct, whereas the inferior division innervates the crista of the posterior semicircular duct and the macula of the saccule.[12] The vestibular nerve travels with the cochlear nerve to form CN VIII. The vestibulocochlear nerve is enclosed in a common sheath of dura mater with the facial nerve as they pass through the internal acoustic meatus. The vestibular nuclei in the brainstem process this information and send messages to the rest of the body to keep the animal upright (facilitatory effect on the ipsilateral extensor muscles of the limb via the vestibulospinal tract). Messages are also sent to the muscles controlling movement of the eyes via medial longitudinal fasciculus and CNs III, IV, and VI to change the position of the eyes according to the position of the head. This way, the visual system can compensate for movements while keeping images stable in the retina.

Cochlea

The cochlea is the coiled part of the membranous labyrinth that is embedded within the rostral portion of the petrous portion of the temporal bone. It is the portion of the inner ear involved in hearing via the cochlear nerve. The fluid-filled cochlea contains the organ of Corti, which is located on the basilar membrane and traverses the length of the structure. The cochlea's role is to transduce sound waves transmitted by the tympanum and the chain of three auditory ossicles (malleus, incus, and stapes) to action potentials of CN VIII. Acoustic pressure waves in the cochlea cause the basilar membrane to vibrate, leading to electrical changes across the membrane of the receptor cells of the organ of Corti. The neurons forming the cochlear branch of CN VIII have their cell bodies in the spiral ganglion of CN VIII. They receive impulses from the neuroepithelial hair cells of the organ of Corti, enter the brainstem, and synapse with the cochlear nuclei. The auditory information is then transmitted to the contralateral medial geniculate nucleus of the diencephalon via the lateral lemniscus. From this nucleus, a third neuron projects via the auditory radiation to the contralateral auditory cortex. Further information can be found in the articles by Ryugo and Strain elsewhere in this issue.

NEUROLOGIC MANIFESTATIONS OF EAR DISEASE
Facial Nerve Paralysis

Clinical presentation

Facial nerve paralysis commonly accompanies middle and inner ear disease, especially otitis media (**Fig. 2**).[3] As it runs in the petrosal portion of the temporal bone, the facial canal that is adjacent to the tympanic cavity lacks a bony wall for a very short distance (**Fig. 3**). This leaves the facial nerve exposed to the cavity and, therefore, to disease processes affecting the middle ear.[13] A lesion at this level causes complete facial paresis or paralysis. Motor dysfunction of CN VII produces ipsilateral drooping of and inability to move the ear and lip, a widened palpebral fissure and absent spontaneous and provoked blinking, absent abduction of the nostril during inspiration, and deviation of the nose toward the normal side due to the unopposed muscle tone on the unaffected side.[14] Provided that normal tear flow is present (unaffected parasympathetic supply of the lacrimal gland), distribution of the corneal film is maintained because passive third eyelid movement by retraction of the globe (mediated by CN VI) is unaffected. With chronic denervation, the lips are retracted farther than normal and the nostril is deviated to the affected side as a result of muscle fibrosis.

Facial spasm can also be seen, causing retraction of the lips and nostril to the affected side, and narrowing of the palpebral fissure on the affected side. This can be distinguished from chronic denervation by performing the palpebral test: in facial spasm the eye can blink. A primary irritation of the facial nerve nucleus, irritation of the lower motor neuron, or increased excitability of the facial nucleus by upper motor neuron dysfunction may cause a constant state of contraction of the ipsilateral facial muscle. This is described as hemifacial spasm. The spasm has been reported early in

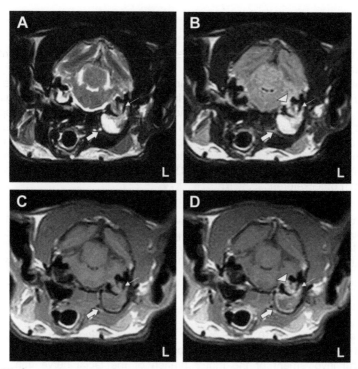

Fig. 2. MRIs from a 10-year-old female neutered domestic short-hair cat that that presented with a 12-week history of acute onset left-sided peripheral vestibular signs (left-sided head tilt and positional horizontal nystagmus) and facial nerve paralysis. Transverse MRIs (*A–D*) are taken at the level of the tympanic bullae and inner ear. Mixed signal intensity material is seen within the left tympanic bulla (*white block arrow*) on T2-weighted (*A*) and FLAIR (*B*) images that is isointense to gray matter on T1-weighted precontrast (*C*) images with peripheral rim contrast enhancement following administration of intravenous paramagnetic contrast medium (*D*). There is a loss of the normal high signal from the left inner ear compared with the right on T2-weighted images (*white line arrows*). The left vestibulocochlear nerve is thickened and is hyperintense to gray matter on FLAIR images (*A*) and the adjacent meninges in this region (*white arrow head*) are also hyperintense on FLAIR images with contrast enhancement on T1-weighted postcontrast images (*C*). These imaging features were compatible with otitis media and/or interna with intracranial extension. (*Courtesy of* Dr L.S. Garosi and Mr M.L. Lowrie, Davies Veterinary Specialists, Higham Gobion, UK.)

the course of middle ear diseases and preceding facial paralysis in some cases, with chronic otitis media,[15,16] and in two dogs with an intracranial mass.[17]

Diagnosis

The motor function of CN VII is primarily assessed by observation of the face for symmetry (position of the ears and lip commissure on each side within the same plane, symmetry of the palpebral fissure), spontaneous blinking, and movement of the nostrils. It also is the motor response (efferent part) of following tests: palpebral reflex, corneal reflex, menace response, and pinching of the face.[14] The parasympathetic supply of the lacrimal gland associated with CN VII can be evaluated by the Schirmer tear test strips. This test quantitatively assesses the tear flow by measuring the distance a fluid line moves on a piece of filter paper inserted in the lower conjunctival fornix at the outer half of the palpebral fissure. In normal dogs and cats, tear

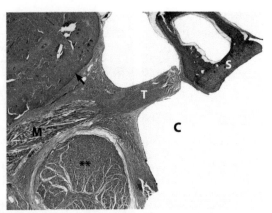

Fig. 3. Histologic section of the stapes, stapedius muscle, and facial nerve of a cat. The facial nerve (*double asterisk*) is in the facial canal. In this section, the bony canal is incomplete, exposing the facial nerve to the tympanic cavity (C). The stapedius muscle (M) is clearly visible in this section with its tendon (T) attached to the head of the tangentially sectioned stapes (S). Bony margin of the petrous portion of the temporal bone (*arrow*). Hematoxylin-eosin stain. (*Courtesy of* Dr B.L. Njaa, Center for Veterinary Health Sciences, Oklahoma State University, Columbus, OH.)

production ranges from 10 to 25 mm in 1 minute. Salivation can be subjectively assessed by examining the mouth for a moist mucosa.

Unilateral involvement of the motor branch of the facial nerve can be seen when asymmetry of the ears, eyelids, lips, and nose are observed. Dysfunction of the parasympathetic supply of the lacrimal gland produces neurogenic keratoconjunctivitis sicca. Affected animals may have recurrent corneal ulceration, mucous discharge from the eye, conjunctival hyperemia, and chronic keratitis. This is mainly seen with lesions of the portion of the facial nerve located between the medulla and the middle ear. Lesions distal to the facial canal in the temporal bone will not affect the parasympathetic division of the facial nerve.[10]

Differential diagnosis

Facial nerve paralysis can be seen with a myriad of conditions, including middle ear disease (eg, infection, polyps, tumors), head trauma and/or peripheral nerve trauma, intracranial neoplasms (eg, meningioma), hypothyroidism, use of potentiated sulfonamides (hypersensitivity), as part of a polyneuropathy, or as an idiopathic condition. The latter is the most common cause of facial nerve paralysis (75% of dogs and 25% of cats).[18,19] The diagnosis of idiopathic facial nerve paralysis is made by exclusion of other possible causes. Facial paralysis is the most common neurologic complication following total ear canal ablation lateral bulla osteotomy (TECA LBO) in dogs (13%–36% of procedures).[20–27] The incidence of facial paralysis in cats following TECA LBO is reported to be considerably higher (as many as 74% procedures) than in dogs.[20,25,28]

Management

Management of facial nerve paralysis consists of treatment of the underlying cause, if one is identified, and management of secondary clinical effects of facial denervation. The main focus should be on preventing the development of a corneal lesion. Corneal keratitis and/or ulcerations may ultimately occur due to exposure associated with the lack of eyelid closure or to the inefficient and/or absent production of tears (involvement of the proximal portion of the facial nerve affecting the parasympathetic general visceral efferent component). Therefore, the cornea needs to be prophylactically lubricated using artificial tears. The prognosis of facial nerve paralysis varies depending on the underlying cause. When secondary to otitis media, many animals make a gradual recovery over a few weeks to months, whereas others will be left with permanent deficits. These deficits may progress to produce muscle contracture and deform facial expression permanently. Most facial nerve paralysis following TECA LBO is temporary and fully resolves within several weeks in dogs, whereas 20% to 47% of procedures result in permanent facial nerve paralysis in cats.[20,25,28] In general, animals that present with facial nerve paralysis before surgery do not show improvement after the procedure.[27]

Vestibular Syndrome

Middle and inner ear disease can result in peripheral vestibular syndrome secondary to involvement of the vestibular receptors in the inner ear and vestibulocochlear nerve. Facial nerve paralysis and/or HS can be seen in association with the vestibular signs, due to the close association of CN VII (facial nerve) and the oculosympathetic supply within the petrous temporal bone. These signs are usually unilateral and ipsilateral to the diseased ear and, on occasion, present bilaterally. Finally, central, instead of, peripheral vestibular signs can predominate in rare cases of otogenic intracranial infection or extension of middle or inner ear neoplasia to the brainstem.

Clinical presentation

Vestibular disease may result in any or all of the following clinical signs: head tilt, ataxia, falling, leaning, rolling, circling, spontaneous or positional nystagmus, and positional strabismus.[29,30]

Head tilt is described as a rotation of the median plane of the head along the axis of the body resulting in one ear being held lower than the other ear. It occurs in vestibular dysfunction as a result of the loss of antigravity muscle tone on one side of the neck. It must be differentiated from a head turn in which the median plane of the head remains perpendicular to the ground but the nose is turned to one side.[14] A head turn is usually associated with a body turn (pleurothotonus) and circling. It does not indicate a vestibular disorder and is usually toward the side of a forebrain lesion.

Nystagmus is an involuntary rhythmic movement of the eyeballs. Physiologic (or vestibular) nystagmus is a nystagmus that occurs in normal animals, whereas pathologic nystagmus reflects an underlying vestibular disorder. In both instances, the nystagmus has a slow and fast phase (ie, jerk nystagmus). A physiologic nystagmus can be induced in normal individuals by rotation of the head from side to side (oculovestibular reflex). This is best performed on a cat by holding the animal at arm's length and rotating it from side to side. This nystagmus stabilizes images on the retina during head movement. It is always observed in the plane of rotation of the head and consists of a slow phase in the direction opposite to that of the head rotation with a fast phase in the same direction as the head rotation. In the absence of any head movement, nystagmus should never be present in a normal animal. Two types of pathologic nystagmus can be observed with vestibular disorders: spontaneous (observed when the head is in a normal position at rest) and positional, which occurs when the head is held in different positions (eg, to either side, dorsally, or by placing the animal upside down on its back).[30] Nystagmus is usually classified based on its direction (the fast movement) and may be horizontal, vertical, or rotatory. By convention, the direction of the nystagmus is described according to the direction of its fast phase. This can be confusing because the lesion is present on the side of the slow phase of the nystagmus (ie, a horizontal nystagmus with the fast phase to the right side indicates a left-sided lesion of the vestibular system).

Positional strabismus can be seen associated with vestibular dysfunction when the head is placed in an abnormal position (extended dorsally or the animal placed upside down on its back). Vestibular dysfunction often causes a ventral or ventrolateral positional strabismus in the eye ipsilateral to the vestibular lesion.

Ataxia is caused by a lack of vestibular input to the ipsilateral limb extensor muscles. This results in swaying of the trunk and head, leaning, falling, and rolling to one side with a unilateral lesion. The patient may tend to circle toward the affected side. These circles are usually small, which will make it appear as though the patient is falling in that direction.[14] The laterally recumbent animal prefers to lie on the side of the body with the lesion and the ipsilateral limb often has decreased extensor tone.

Other vestibular signs include leaning, falling, and wide-based stance. The vestibular system affects limb tone via the vestibulospinal tract, which facilitates the ipsilateral extensor muscles and inhibits the contralateral extensor muscles. With unilateral vestibular disease, the lack of vestibular input can result in the animal leaning and falling on the affected side as a result of the ipsilateral limb having decreased extensor tone and contralateral limbs having increased extensor tone.[31,32]

All of the above are manifestations of unilateral vestibular disease. Bilateral vestibular disease is characterized by a head sway from side to side, loss of balance on either side, and symmetric ataxia with a crouched posture closer to the ground surface.[30] A physiologic nystagmus usually cannot be elicited and a head tilt is not observed. Bilateral vestibular disease can occur as a result of lesion affecting both peripheral vestibular components (ie, bilateral middle or inner ear disease; **Fig. 4**) or, less commonly, both central vestibular components.

Occasionally, an otogenic infection can extend into the cranial vault causing secondary intracranial epidural empyema, meningoencephalitis, and/or brain abscess (**Fig. 5**). Neoplasms of the middle or inner ear may also progress to involve the brain stem. In these instances, central, instead of peripheral, vestibular signs predominate.[33–35] Associated brainstem signs may be present, including abnormal mental status; ipsilateral upper motor neuron hemiparesis; and/or tetraparesis and general proprioceptive ataxia; and conscious proprioceptive deficits. Associated forebrain signs include epileptic seizures, abnormal behavior, loss of vision, conscious proprioceptive deficits, and facial hypalgesia. The most likely anatomic pathway for entry of organisms from the inner ear into the brainstem of dogs and cats is along the nerves and vessels of the internal acoustic meatus.[36] Not all affected animals present concurrent facial nerve involvement.[36] Cerebrospinal fluid (CSF) analysis may be diagnostically useful, especially in acute or subacute cases. The long-term outcome seems to be good in most cases of intracranial extension of otitis media and/or interna after aggressive surgical and medical therapy.[36]

Diagnosis

Although the vestibular signs associated with ear disease are expected to be peripheral in nature, the clinician should focus on identifying other neurologic signs suggestive of middle and/or inner ear disease and ruling out brainstem involvement.

Facial nerve paralysis and/or HS can be seen concurrently with vestibular signs in an animal with ear disease due to the proximity of CN VII (facial nerve) and the ocular sympathetic nerve supply, with the vestibular nerve in the region of the petrous temporal bone.[30]

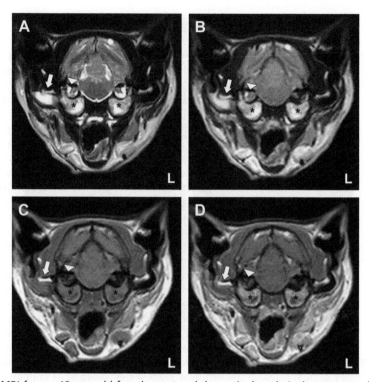

Fig. 4. MRI from a 12-year-old female neutered domestic short hair that presented with a 3-week history of acute onset progressive bilateral peripheral vestibular signs (a marked head sway with vestibular ataxia) and right-sided HS. Transverse MRIs (*A–D*) are taken at the level of the tympanic bullae. Mixed signal intensity material is seen within both tympanic bullae (*black asterisks*) on T2-weighted (*A*) and FLAIR (*B*) images that is isointense to gray matter on T1-weighted precontrast (*C*) images with moderate contrast enhancement following administration intravenous paramagnetic contrast medium (*D*). Nonenhancing and T2-hyperintense material is evident in the right external ear canal (*white arrows*). The right inner ear has an area of decreased signal intensity on T2-weighted images (*white arrow heads*), which fails to suppress on FLAIR but enhances on T1-weighted postcontrast images. These imaging findings are compatible with bilateral otitis media in addition to right-sided otitis externa and interna. (*Courtesy of* Dr L.S. Garosi and Mr M.L. Lowrie, Davies Veterinary Specialists, Higham Gobion, UK.)

Both peripheral and central vestibular disease can cause a head tilt, horizontal or rotatory nystagmus, positional strabismus, and ataxia. Correctly identifying central vestibular disease requires identification of clinical signs that cannot be attributed to diseases of the peripheral vestibular system.[30] Lesions that affect the central vestibular system typically have additional clinical signs suggestive of brainstem involvement. Such lesions often involve the reticular formation as well as ascending and descending motor and sensory pathways to the ipsilateral limbs. Therefore, abnormal mental status (depression, stupor, coma), ipsilateral upper motor neuron hemiparesis and general proprioceptive ataxia, and conscious proprioceptive deficits are commonly associated with central vestibular disease. Deficits of CNs V through XII (other than VII and VIII) can also be associated with central vestibular disease. The presence of spontaneous or positional jerk nystagmus indicates vestibular disease

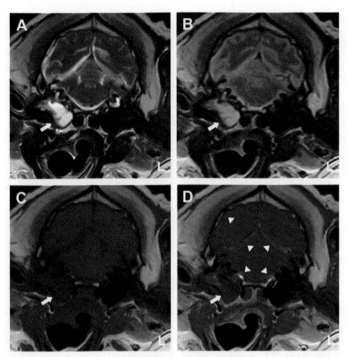

Fig. 5. MRI scan from a 9-year-old female neutered Bassett hound that presented with a 48-hour history of right-sided central vestibular signs (a right-sided head tilt, obtundation and right-sided proprioceptive deficits) and pyrexia. Transverse MRIs (*A–E*) taken at the level of the tympanic bullae and inner ear reveal a thickening of the external ear canal with hyperintense material seen within the right tympanic bulla (*white block arrow*) on T2-weighted (*A*) and FLAIR (*B*) image. This material is isointense to gray matter on T1-weighted precontrast (*C*) images with peripheral rim contrast enhancement following administration intravenous paramagnetic contrast medium (*D*). Subtraction maneuver (*E*) highlighting areas of contrast enhancement. The ventral subarachnoid space at the level of the rostral medulla oblongata appears widened on the T2-weighted (*A*) image and is hyperintense to gray matter on FLAIR (*B*) images. There is evidence of meningeal contrast enhancement in this region, around the tentorium cerebelli and surrounding the forebrain (*D; white arrow heads*). These changes are clearly highlighted using a subtraction maneuver (*E*). These imaging features are compatible with otitis media/interna with intracranial extension. Cerebrospinal fluid (CSF) collected from the cerebellomedullary cistern was xanthochromic and extremely turbid. Cytology revealed mixed inflammatory cells, scattered erythrocytes, small free proliferating diplococcoid bacteria (*F; white arrow heads*) and phagocytosed bacteria (*F; white arrow*). The nucleated cells are primarily neutrophils with low numbers of small reactive lymphocytes and vacuolated macrophages. The neutrophils are observed on occasion to phagocytose the bacteria with intracytoplasmic chains of bacteria seen (*G; white arrow*). The protein concentration was 475 mg/dL (normal <30). Culture of the CSF yielded a moderate growth of beta-hemolytic *Streptococcus pneumoniae* after 48-hour incubation. The dog underwent a right-sided total ear canal ablation and lateral bulla ostectomy. The tympanic membrane was found to be ruptured at the time of surgery. A 4-week course of metronidazole (10 mg/kg every 12 hours by mouth) and cephalexin (20 mg/kg twice a day by mouth) was given and the dog made a good and complete recovery. (*A–E*) *Courtesy of* Dr L.S. Garosi and Mr M.L. Lowrie, Davies Veterinary Specialists, Higham Gobion, UK. (*F–G*) *Courtesy of* Mr R. Powell, Powell Torrance Diagnostic Services, Higham Gobion, UK.)

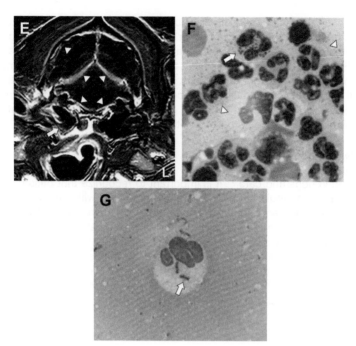

Fig. 5. (*continued*)

but does not further localize the lesion to the peripheral or central vestibular system. However, vertical nystagmus and nystagmus that change in direction on change position of the head (ie, variable nystagmus) are a feature of central vestibular lesions.[14] The rate of nystagmus (number of beats per minute [BPM] with the head in a neutral position and with the animal in dorsal recumbency) can further assist with differentiation between central vestibular disease and peripheral disease according to a study by Troxel and colleagues[35] (2005). The median rate of resting and positional nystagmus seems significantly faster for dogs with peripheral vestibular disease—with a resting nystagmus greater than or equal to 66 BPM. This observation provides the highest combined sensitivity and specificity in diagnosing peripheral vestibular disease. In this study, a rate of resting nystagmus greater than 66 BPM was associated with high sensitivity (85%) and specificity (95%) for diagnosis of peripheral vestibular syndrome.

If in doubt about the localization of the lesion, the clinician should investigate the animal for central vestibular disease as well as peripheral vestibular disease.[14] Advanced diagnostic imaging is essential in evaluating patients with clinical evidence of central vestibular disease or if in doubt about the location of the neurologic lesion. CT scan and MRI are complimentary imaging techniques of the middle and inner ear. Although a CT scan can be used to better define bony structures, MRI allows distinction of soft tissues components, including intralabyrinthine fluid, CSF, nerves, and vessels within the internal auditory canal, as well as meninges and brain parenchyma.[37] It is, therefore, the authors' preferred imaging modality to investigate vestibular disorders associated with ear disease. Aside from helping in the diagnosis of middle ear disease, MRI allows the structures within the petrous portion of the temporal bone to be delineated and various pathologic lesions of the membranous labyrinth to be detected.[37–39] T2-weighted images enable visualization of intralabyrinthine fluid in the semicircular ducts and cochlea. In chronic otitis interna, fibrous obliteration of the fluid-containing spaces of the inner ear may occur and can be detected by the absence of signal in T2-weighted images on the affected side (see **Fig. 2**).[37] Contrast enhancement may also be seen inside the membranous labyrinth in the acute phase of labyrinthitis.[37] In the case of central vestibular involvement, MRI is the imaging modality of choice, especially with regard to evaluating the caudal fossa.[40] CSF should be collected because it may be diagnostically useful, especially in acute or subacute cases of otogenic intracranial infection.[36]

Differential diagnosis
Otitis media and/or interna are the most common causes of peripheral vestibular disease seen in dogs and cats.[41] It is important to recognize that otitis media alone will not result in vestibular signs. If deficits compatible with peripheral vestibular dysfunction are detected, inner ear involvement is confirmed.[29] Other causes of peripheral vestibular disorder include hypothyroidism, aural neoplasia, nasopharyngeal and otopharyngeal polyps, ototoxicity (especially aminoglycoside antibiotics, topical iodophors, or topical chlorhexidine), and acute idiopathic peripheral vestibular disease.[30] Vestibular syndrome may also be iatrogenic following bulla osteotomy in 3% to 8% of dogs.[20,22,23,42] It can also predate the surgery as a result of pressure on labyrinthine structures due to accumulation of polyp or mucous material with the tympanic cavitiy.[43]

Management
Treatment of a vestibular disorder consists primarily in treating the underlying cause. Meclizine (12.5 mg by mouth every 12 hours in dogs; 6.25 mg by mouth every 12 hours in cats), diazepam (0.1–0.5 mg/kg by mouth every 8 hours in dogs; 1–2 mg by mouth every 12 hours in cats) and/or maropitant (1 mg/kg subcutaneous every 24 hours or 2 mg/kg by mouth every 24 hours in dogs) are sometimes helpful in decreasing signs associated with an acute vestibular disorder. These signs include nausea and anorexia, as well as, in some instances, the severity of the head tilt and ataxia.[30] The prognosis is good for resolution of the infection in cases of otitis media and/or interna, but neurologic deficits such as a mild head tilt and mild ataxia may persist despite effective therapy because of permanent damage to neural structures. The presence of persistent nystagmus is suggestive of an active disease process.[30] Head tilt and vestibular signs that persist longer than 2 to 3 weeks are usually permanent or improve incompletely over time.[20,23,42,43]

In case of otogenic intracranial infection, antibiotic selection should be based on culture or sensitivity results obtained from the middle ear following surgical drainage of the tympanic cavity and/or CSF sampling, if available.[36] Antibiotic selection should additionally be based on an antibiotic that effectively crosses the blood-brain or CSF barrier. Empiric antibiotics should initially be given intravenously for 2 to 3 days to reach therapeutic levels in a timely manner. The authors use trimethoprim sulfonamide (30 to 60 mg/kg every 24 hours), metronidazole (10–15 mg/kg every 12 hours), cefuroxime (10–15 mg/kg every 8 hours), or enrofloxacin (5–10 mg/kg every 24 hours). Antibiotics should be continued for 3 to 4 weeks after clinical signs have resolved. Intravenous mannitol (0.2–2 g/kg slow bolus over 10–20 minutes every 4–6 hours as needed) and/or dexamethasone (0.05–0.1 mg/kg every 24 hours for the first 24–48 hours) can be given to reduce vasogenic brain edema and an associated increase in intracranial pressure. Surgical drainage and decompression by craniectomy or burr holes may be indicated in cases of subdural intracranial empyema.

HS

Clinical presentation

The loss of sympathetic innervation to the eye causes a combination of clinical signs that are collectively termed HS. This syndrome manifests as a quartet of clinical signs[9,44]:

- Miosis
- Drooping of the upper eyelid (ptosis) due to loss of smooth muscle tone affecting the Müller muscle
- Enophthalmos, caused by combined effects of denervation of the orbital smooth muscles that fill the periorbita, and the antagonist action of the extraocular muscles (especially the retractor bulbi muscles), causing retraction of the eyeball
- Protrusion of the third eyelid due to denervation of the smooth muscle of the eyelid and concurrent enophthalmos resulting in passive protraction of the third eyelid.

HS is most often seen in animals with diseases of the middle ear[3,44] or after surgery of the ear canal.[21,24,25] HS can be present as a sole neurologic manifestation or associated with facial nerve paralysis and/or peripheral vestibular disorder.

Diagnosis

A lesion anywhere along the three-neuron ocular sympathetic pathway can cause HS. HS is classified according to the level of the lesion along the sympathetic pathway as first (upper motor neuron), second (preganglionic fibers), or third order (postganglionic fibers). Therefore, lesions causing HS tend to affect a region as opposed to a specific nucleus or nerve and, therefore, accompanying neurologic signs are useful to further locate a lesion within the sympathetic pathway. This syndrome is most commonly seen with lesions affecting the preganglionic fibers located within the intermediate gray matter of the T1 to T3 spinal cord segments to the tympanic bulla and the postganglionic fibers located between the tympanic bulla and the eye. In addition to the presence and development of accompanying neurologic signs, pharmacologic testing can help to localize the site of the lesion. A direct-acting sympathomimetic drug, 1% to 10% phenylephrine, is administered topically to both eyes and the time taken for the pupils to dilate is noted. If the lesion is postganglionic (third order HS), as can be seen with middle ear disease, the sympathetically innervated iris sphincter muscle becomes supersensitive to direct acting sympathomimetics and, thus, responds to subpharmacological and ordinarily ineffective concentrations of phenylephrine. In that instance, topical administration of one drop of 1% phenylephrine leads to mydriasis in the affected eye within 20 minutes.[45] If 10% phenylephrine is used, mydriasis occurs in 5 to 8 minutes.[46]

Differential diagnosis

HS secondary to middle ear disease should be differentiated from other causes of third order HS, such as middle cranial fossa pathologic abnormalities (neoplasm, vascular anomalies, infection), retrobulbar pathologic abnormalities (contusion, abscess or neoplasm), and idiopathic HS. The latter is the most common cause of third order HS.[8,47] HS can also been seen as complication of surgery for middle ear disease and especially ventral bulla osteotomy in cats.[20,25,28] It has been reported in as much as 53% of cases in one study with most cases (46%) being temporary.[25] This complication can be associated with the concurrent development of peripheral vestibular signs. It is usually the result of either the osteotomy or overzealous curettage. Signs of HS usually resolve in the course of a few days. When signs persist beyond 6 weeks, patients are unlikely to recover fully.[43]

Management

Management of HS consists primarily in treating the underlying cause. Topical 10% phenylephrine can be used to provide occasional, short-term alleviation of the signs if vision is obscured by the third eyelid protrusion.[46]

SUMMARY

Diseases affecting the ear can be broadly divided into inflammatory and noninflammatory conditions. Otitis and neoplasia represent the main differential diagnoses.

Because the facial and sympathetic nerves course near the middle ear, a facial nerve paralysis and/or HS may occur on the same side as the middle ear disease.

The clinical signs of inner ear disease in the dog and cat are usually those of a peripheral vestibular syndrome, which reflect injury to the vestibular nerve or receptor organs.

Although deafness may also be caused by inner ear disease, it may not be clinically noticeable with unilateral involvement.

REFERENCES

1. Getty R, Foust HL, Prestley ET, et al. Macroscopic anatomy of the ear of the dog. Am J Vet Res 1956;17:364–75.
2. Evans HE. The ear. In: Evans HE, editor. Miller's Anatomy of the dog. 3rd edition. Philadelphia: WB Saunders; 1993. p. 731–45.
3. Cook LB. Neurologic evaluation of the ear. Vet Clin North Am Small Anim Pract 2004;34:425–35.
4. King AS. Nuclei of the cranial nerves. In: King AS, editor. Physiological and clinical anatomy of the domestic mammals. Oxford (United Kingdom): Oxford University Press; 1987. p. 79–80.
5. Whalen LR, Kitchell RL. Electrophysiological studies of the cutaneous nerves of the head of the dog. Am J Vet Res 1983;44:615–27.
6. Evans HE. The skeleton. In: Evans HE, editor. Miller's Anatomy of the dog. 3rd edition. Philadelphia: WB Saunders; 1993.
7. Evans HE, Kitchell RL. Cranial nerves and cutaneous innervation of the head. In: Evans HE, editor. Miller's Anatomy of the dog. 3rd edition. Philadelphia: WB Saunders; 1993. p. 708–30.
8. Neer TM. Horner's syndrome: anatomy, diagnosis, and causes. Comp Cont Educ Pract Vet 1984;6:740–6.
9. Van Den Broek AH. Horner's syndrome in cats and dogs: a review. J Small Anim Pract 1987;28:929–40.
10. de Lahunta A, Glass E. Lower motor neuron: general visceral efferent system. Veterinary neuroanatomy and clinical neurology. 3rd edition. St Louis (MO): WB Saunders Co; 2009. p. 168–91.
11. Cunningham JG, Klein BG. The vestibular system. In: Cunningham JG, Klein BG, editors. Textbook of veterinary physiology. 4th edition. St Louis (MO): Saunders Elsevier; 2007.
12. Blauch B, Strafuss AC. Histologic relationship of the facial (7th) and vestibulocochlear (8th) cranial nerves within the petrous temporal bone in the dog. Am J Vet Res 1974;35:481–6.

13. de Lahunta A, Glass E. Lower motor neuron: general somatic efferent, cranial nerve. Veterinary neuroanatomy and clinical neurology. 3rd edition. St Louis (MO): WB Saunders Co; 2009. p. 134–67.
14. Garosi LS. Neurological examination. In: Platt SR, Olby NJ, editors. BSAVA Manual of canine and feline neurology. 3rd edition. Quedgeley (United Kingdom): BSAVA; 2004. p. 1–23.
15. Roberts SR, Vainisi SJ. Hemifacial spasm in dogs. J Am Vet Med Assoc 1967; 150:381–5.
16. Parker AJ, Cusick PK, Park RD, et al. Hemifacial spasms in a dog. Vet Rec 1973; 93:514–6.
17. Van Meervenne SA, Bhatti SF, Martlé V, et al. Hemifacial spasm associated with an intracranial mass in two dogs. J Small Anim Pract 2008;48:472–5.
18. Braund KG, Luttgen PJ, Sorjonen DC, et al. Idiopathic facial paralysis in the dog. Vet Rec 1979;105:297–9.
19. Kern TJ, Erb HN. Facial neuropathy in dogs and cats: 95 cases (1975–1985). J Am Vet Med Assoc 1987;191:1604–9.
20. Smeak DD, Dehoff WD. Total ear canal ablation: clinical results in the dog and cat. Vet Surg 1986;15:161–70.
21. Boothe HW. Surgical management of otitis media and otitis interna. Vet Clin North Am Small Anim Pract 1988;18:901–11.
22. Mason LK, Harvey CE, Orsher RJ. Total ear canal ablation combined with lateral bulla osteotomy for end-stage otitis in dogs. Results in thirty dogs. Vet Surg 1988; 17:263–8.
23. White RA, Pomeroy CJ. Total ear canal ablation and lateral bulla osteotomy in the dog. J Small Anim Pract 1990;31:547–53.
24. Trevor PB, Martin RA. Tympanic bulla osteotomy for treatment of middle-ear disease in cats: 19 cases (1984-1991). J Am Vet Med Assoc 1993;202:123–9.
25. Bacon NJ, Gilbert RL, Bostock DE, et al. Total ear canal ablation in the cat: indications, morbidity and long-term survival. J Small Anim Pract 2003;44:430–4.
26. Doust R, King A, Hammond G, et al. Assessment of middle ear disease in the dog: a comparison of diagnostic imaging modalities. J Small Anim Pract 2007; 48:188–92.
27. Smeak DD. Management of complications associated with total ear canal ablation and bulla osteotomy in dogs and cats. Vet Clin North Am Small Anim Pract 2011;41:981–94.
28. Williams JM, White RA. Total ear canal ablation combined with lateral bulla osteotomy in the cat. J Small Anim Pract 1992;33:225–7.
29. Rossmeisl H Jr. Vestibular disease in dogs and cats. Vet Clin North Am Small Anim Pract 2010;40:81–100.
30. Garosi LS. (2012) Head tilt and nystagmus. In: Platt SR, Garosi LS, editors. Small animal neurological emergencies. 1st edition. Manson; 2012. p. 253–63.
31. de Lahunta A, Glass E. Vestibular system: special proprioception. Veterinary neuroanatomy and clinical neurology. 3rd edition. St Louis (MO): WB Saunders Co; 2009.
32. de Lahunta A, Glass E. Auditory system: special somatic afferent system. Veterinary neuroanatomy and clinical neurology. 3rd edition. St Louis (MO): WB Saunders Co; 2009.
33. Klopp LS, Hathcock JT, Sorjonen DC. Magnetic resonance imaging features of brain stem abscessation in two cats. Vet Radiol Ultrasound 2000;41:300–7.
34. Spangler EA, Dewey CW. Meningoencephalitis secondary to bacterial otitis media/interna in a dog. J Am Anim Hosp Assoc 2000;36:239–43.

35. Troxel MT, Drobatz KJ, Vite CH. Signs of neurological dysfunction in dogs with central versus peripheral vestibular disease. J Am Vet Med Assoc 2005;227: 570–4.

36. Sturges BK, Dickinson PJ, Kortz GD, et al. Clinical signs, magnetic resonance imaging features, and outcome after surgical and medical treatment of otogenic intracranial infection in 11 cats and 4 dogs. J Vet Intern Med 2006;20:648–56.

37. Garosi LS, Dennis R, Schwarz T. Review of diagnostic imaging of ear diseases in the dog and cat. Vet Radiol Ultrasound 2003;44:137–46.

38. Dvir E, Kirberger RM, Terblanche AG. Magnetic resonance imaging of otitis interna in a dog. Vet Radiol Ultrasound 2000;41:46–9.

39. Garosi LS, Lamb CR, Targett MP. Magnetic resonance imaging findings in a dog with otitis media and suspected otitis interna. Vet Record 2000;146:501–2.

40. Garosi LS, Dennis R, Penderis J, et al. Results of magnetic resonance imaging in dogs with vestibular disorders: 85 cases (1996–1999). J Am vet Med Assoc 2001; 218:385–91.

41. Shunk KL, Averill DR. Peripheral vestibular syndrome in the dog: a review of 83 cases. J Am Vet Med Assoc 1983;182:1354–7.

42. Matthieson DT, Scavelli T. Total ear canal ablation and lateral bulla osteotomy in 38 dogs. J Am Anim Hosp Assoc 1990;26:257–67.

43. White RA. Middle ear. In: Slatter D, editor. Textbook of small animal surgery. 3rd edition. Philadelphia: Saunders, Elsevier Science; 2003. p. 1757–67.

44. Kern TJ, Aromando MC, Erb HN. Horner's syndrome in dogs and cats: 100 cases (1975–1985). J Am Vet Med Assoc 1989;195:369–73.

45. Bistner SI, Rubin LF, Cox TA, et al. Pharmacologic diagnosis of Horner's syndrome in the dog. J Am Vet Med Assoc 1970;157:1220–4.

46. Penderis J. Disorders of the eyes and vision. In: Platt SR, Olby NJ, editors. BSAVA Manual of canine and feline neurology. 3rd edition. Quedgeley (United Kingdom): BSAVA; 2004. p. 133–54.

47. Boydell P. Idiopathic Horner's syndrome in the golden retriever. J Small Anim Pract 1995;36:382–4.

Tumors and Tumorlike Lesions of Dog and Cat Ears

Mee Ja M. Sula, DVM

KEYWORDS

- Ear • Neoplasia • Otitis

KEY POINTS

- Although uncommon, neoplasia of the auricular structures is an important cause of otic and central nervous system–associated morbidity and mortality and should be considered possible in any case of nonresponsive otitis.
- The frequent association of chronic otitis with neoplastic transformation of auricular components underlies the importance of early and aggressive treatment of inflammatory ear disease.
- Numerous otic entities present with similar clinical histories and examination findings and advanced diagnostics including histopathology, cytology, and imaging are essential investigative tools.

INTRODUCTION

Patients presenting with auricular disease commonly exhibit a wide spectrum of symptoms including otorrhea, otorrhagia, otalgia, head shaking, scratching, odor, loss of hearing, facial nerve paralysis, pain on opening the mouth, and vestibular signs. In most cases, chronic and ongoing otitis provides a functional explanation for these clinical signs; however, less commonly, these signs are indicatory of a space-occupying lesion within the auricular structures. A broad array of space-occupying nonneoplastic, benign, and malignant neoplasms may localize to the ear (**Box 1**). The ear's involvement in such an immense array of disease processes is partially explained by the vastly different anatomic and histologic features of the component auricular structures (discussed elsewhere in this issue). Inflammatory or neoplastic disease may be centered on or arise from any one of several tissue types including epithelial (overlying epidermis, adnexal structures, membranes lining middle and internal ear structures); mesenchymal (dermis, auricular cartilage, bone, muscle); or nervous tissue.

The author has nothing to disclose.
Department of Veterinary Pathobiology, Center for Veterinary Health Sciences, Oklahoma State University, 250 McElroy Hall, Stillwater, OK 74078, USA
E-mail address: mee-ja.sula@okstate.edu

Vet Clin Small Anim 42 (2012) 1161–1178
http://dx.doi.org/10.1016/j.cvsm.2012.08.004
0195-5616/12/$ – see front matter

Box 1
Lesions of the ear

Nonneoplastic and benign lesions external ear

- Canine leproid granuloma
- Infectious cutaneous granulomatous diseases
  - Leishmania
  - Sporotrichosis
  - Cryptococcus
  - Opportunistic fungal infections
- Chronic proliferative otitis externa
- Para-auricular abscess
- Adnexal hyperplasia
  - Ceruminous hyperplasia
  - Sebaceous hyperplasia
- Noninfectious cutaneous granulomatous diseases
  - Foreign body
  - Sterile granuloma/pyogranuloma complex
  - Cutaneous xanthoma
  - Canine sarcoid
  - Eosinophilic granuloma complex
  - Langerhans cell histiocytosis
- Follicular cysts
- Apocrine cysts
- Feline ceruminous cystomatosis
- Proliferative and necrotizing otitis (cats)
- Auricular chondritis
- Auricular hematoma
- Cutaneous lymphocytosis
- Psoriasifrom lichenoid dermatosis of English springer spaniels
- Idiopathic, benign lichenoid keratosis
- Actinic keratosis
- Hemangioma
- Canine cutaneous histiocytoma
- Plasmacytoma
- Papilloma (warts)
- Feline cowpox
- Adnexal adenomas
  - Ceruminous gland adenoma
  - Sebaceous gland adenoma
  - Apocrine cystadenoma

- Melanocytoma
- Basal cell tumor
- Rhabdomyoma
- Mast cell tumor

Malignant neoplasm external ear

- Squamous cell carcinoma
- Hemangiosarcoma
- Adnexal carcinoma
  - Ceruminous gland adenocarcinoma
  - Sebaceous gland epithelioma
  - Sebaceous gland adenocarcinoma
- Undifferentiated carcinoma
- Feline sarcoid/fibropapilloma
- Melanoma
- Fibrosarcoma
- Lymphoma
- Granular cell tumor

Nonneoplastic and benign neoplastic lesions middle and internal ear

- Aural cholesteatoma (Aural keratinizing cyst)
- Cholesterol granuloma
- Inflammatory nasopharyngeal polyps
- Craniomandibular osteopathy
- Papillary adenoma

Malignant neoplasms middle and internal ear

- Squamous cell carcinoma
- Undifferentiated adenocarcinoma
- Fibrosarcoma
- Lymphoma

Diagnosis and treatment of space-occupying lesions in the ear are frequently complicated by concurrent disease, typically bacterial and fungal (yeast) infections. This association is not considered coincidental and chronic and ongoing low-grade inflammation can eventually result in hyperplastic or dysplastic changes that predispose to eventual neoplastic transformation. This direct association most commonly involves cutaneous and adnexal structures of the external ear, and in cats is typified by frequent episodes of ear mite infestation and eventual development of ceruminous gland adenocarcinomas.[1] Additionally, development of hyperplastic or neoplastic masses frequently results in partial or complete obstruction of the ear canal, impairing removal of debris, resulting in prolonged and continuous contact with cerumen, postulated by some to be carcinogenic.[1]

Clinical signs, gross, and even radiographic appearances of chronic otitis and neoplasia can be similar; therefore, advanced imaging, cytologic, and histopathologic examination of masses within the ear are essential diagnostic tools. Because the presence of bilateral disease does not rule out neoplasia, neoplasia or other space-occupying lesion should be considered in any case of proliferative, unilateral, or bilateral aural pathology. This article discusses selected features of common and rare neoplastic and nonneoplastic space-occupying lesions of the external, middle, and internal ear.

NONNEOPLASTIC DISEASES: INFECTIOUS AND INFLAMMATORY
Canine Leproid Granuloma (Canine Leprosy)

Leproid granulomas typically present as one to multiple, discreet, nodular, dermal or subcutaneous, pyogranulomatous inflammatory masses caused by an as yet unidentified species of mycobacteria. Lesions have a predilection for the base of the ears, particularly in short-coated breeds of dogs, and are especially frequent in boxer and boxer-cross dogs.[2] Lesions may also occur elsewhere on the head and distal limbs, but lymph node involvement or systemic disease has not been reported. Given the primarily affected locations and propensity for short-coated breeds, infection by this likely saprophytic mycobacterium is thought to be by biting insects or direct, traumatic inoculation. Reported occurrence is more frequent in colder months and, paired with the preferential location to the pinna, may reflect a need for a cooler local environment to facilitate development of these lesions.[2]

Diagnosis is based on identifying the presence of acid-fast bacteria either through fine-needle aspirate cytology or histopathology. Although spontaneous resolution in immunocompetent animals has been reported, treatment options include complete surgical excision or long-term systemic antibiotics.[2]

Infectious Cutaneous Granulomatous Diseases

Any number of infectious agents may cause a nodular, granulomatous dermatitis and may include the pinna as part of more generalized disease. *Leishmania* spp, transmitted by the sandfly, has particular predilection for the sparsely haired ears and face[3] but similar clinical or histologic lesions may be seen with *Blastomyces dermatitidis*, *Cryptococcus* spp, *Histoplasma capsulatum*, *Neospora caninum*, *Toxoplasma gondii*, *Trypanosoma cruzi*, *Sporothrix schenchkii*, and other opportunistic fungal agents.

Chronic Proliferative Otitis Externa

Proliferative (obstructive) otitis externa is the end result of chronic otitis in some dogs and cats and is characterized by marked ceruminous gland hypertrophy and hyperplasia, acanthosis, and proliferation of soft tissues resulting in stenosis and obstruction of the external ear canal. Proliferative changes develop in weeks to months typically at the base of the auricle and inside the external ear canal, leading to occlusion of the canal. In the most chronic cases, calcification and ossification of cartilage leads to irreversible obstructive disease.[4] Proliferative and inflammatory changes can extend to and involve the middle ear. Although identification and medical management of the underlying problem should always be the goal for treatment, surgical intervention in the most advanced cases may be considered.

Para-auricular Abscess

Para-aural swelling and fistulation may occur secondary to any cause of ear canal stenosis,[1] and is most commonly seen in cases of obstructive, hyperplastic proliferation secondary to chronically diseased ears. Neoplasia, otitis media, foreign body migration, traumatic ear canal separation, disease involving the petrous portion of the temporal bone, and ear canal/bulla surgery are all associated with development of para-aural abscessation.[5] Given its association with neoplastic disease, it is critical to determine the underlying cause in any patient that presents with a para-aural abscess.

Inflammatory Nasopharyngeal Polyps

These nonneoplastic, inflammatory masses arise from the mucosal lining of the middle ear, auditory (eustachian) tube, or nasopharynx and are the most commonly reported external ear canal mass in cats. Although much less common in dogs, the condition is of similar origin and clinical progression in this species. Polyps typically extend as a single mass through the auditory tube into either the nasopharynx, where it may cause signs of dysphagia or upper respiratory disease, or the middle ear, resulting in signs attributable to middle or inner ear disease including Horner syndrome, and vestibular signs. Masses originating from the middle ear may extend through the tympanic membrane into the external ear canal causing otorrhea, head shaking, and occasionally presenting as a visible mass obstructing the external ear canal. One report of middle ear polyps in a dog describes multiple, small polyps originating from the medial surface of the tympanic membrane,[6] and a similar presentation is reported in a cat with chronic otitis media.[7] Inflammatory polyps are typically unilateral, but bilateral disease has been reported.[6]

The cause of inflammatory polyps is unknown, and chronic inflammation, ascending pharyngeal infection, congenital origin, and association with feline calicivirus have all been implicated.[8,9] Cats are typically younger than 3 years old when diagnosed; however, dogs and cats of any age may be affected. Diagnosis may be made on finding a firm-to-fleshy mass on otoscopic or oral examination. Advanced imaging may be advantageously used to definitively determine site of origin and aid in the identification of early middle ear involvement.

Treatment is either through simple traction avulsion, which is typically sufficient if there is no middle ear involvement, or through a ventral bulla osteotomy, which is associated with a lower recurrence rate but higher postsurgical complications. Polyps of nasopharyngeal origin are less likely to reoccur than ones of middle ear origin.[8] Concurrent otitis media/interna is a common finding and bacterial culture followed by appropriate antibiotic therapy is recommended. Postoperative treatment with prednisolone at anti-inflammatory doses is believed by some to reduce the likelihood of recurrence regardless of surgical method.[8]

Proliferative and Hyperplastic Lesions

Adnexal hyperplasia

Chronically inflamed ears are commonly associated with ceruminous gland hyperplasia, which is manifested as an increase in size, number, and activity of glands within the external ear canal. In a review of 44 cats that underwent total ear canal ablation for ear disease, marked hyperplasia of the ceruminous glands occurred in more than 50% of the histologically examined ears, always in association with chronic otitis externa.[10] The frequent association between chronic otitis and ceruminous gland hyperplasia, and it's implication as a factor in neoplastic transformation, emphasizes the importance of early and aggressive therapeutic management of otitis in dogs and cats.

Nodular sebaceous gland hyperplasia is a common, spontaneous, nonneoplastic lesion accounting for approximately 23% of all nonneoplastic skin masses in dogs.[11] Lesions typically present as yellow-white, papillated nodules and plaques that arise with particular frequency on the dorsal head, ears, face, and legs. Nodular sebaceous hyperplasia has not been associated with chronic inflammatory disease.

NONNEOPLASTIC DISEASES: NONINFECTIOUS
Proliferative and Necrotizing Otitis Externa (of Kittens)

First described in cats less than 1 year of age, this disease entity of unknown cause is reported in cats up to 5 years-old.[12] The clinical presentation is visually distinctive, consisting of dark brown to black, proliferative, often plaquelike coalescing lesions covering the concave surface of the pinnae and often extending into and obstructing the vertical ear canal. Thick exudate and secondary bacterial or yeast otitis externa frequently accompany the lesion. Pruritus and pain are usually minimal, and occur most frequently in cases that have advanced to ulceration. Lesions typically first appear in kittens aged 2 to 6 months and completely and spontaneously regress by 2 years[13]; however, spontaneous resolution does not occur in all cases.[12]

The cause of proliferative and necrotizing otitis externa is unknown, and given the young age of onset, aberrant viral infection has been postulated; however, an association with several common viruses including Feline Immunodeficiency virus (FIV), Feline Leukemia Virus (FeLV), herpesvirus, calicivirus, and papillomavirus has not been made.[12] Recent work has implicated keratinocyte apoptosis induced by epidermal CD3+ T cells as central in the pathogenesis,[14] although the reason these T cells develop has not been established. This pathogenesis is supported by the effective use of topical tacrolimus, a calcineurin inhibitor known to inhibit T cell–mediated keratinocyte apoptosis, in the treatment of this disease.

Given the typical age and distinctive clinical appearance, diagnosis may be made on clinical examination and confirmed with histopathology. In cases of adult cats with a history of recurrent or clinically refractive otitis externa and suggestive gross lesions, this entity should be considered. Topical treatment with 1% tacrolimus has been shown to be effective in as little as 2 weeks, although some animals may need to be treated for months. It is unclear whether treatment with the tacrolimus or spontaneous regression is responsible for eventual resolution.[12]

Aural Cholesteatoma (Aural Keratinizing Cysts)

Aural cholesteatomas are nonneoplastic, cystic structures composed of a central cavity of keratin debris surrounded by keratinizing, stratified squamous epithelium. Although the term "cholesteatoma" is well entrenched in the literature, the histologic picture is that of a keratinizing cyst, and "aural keratinizing cyst" is the preferred terminology. In dogs, these are considered acquired entities, secondary to migration or invagination of stratified squamous epithelium from the external ear canal. These cysts typically develop after rupture of the tympanic membrane, and are reported to occur in 11% of dogs with chronic otitis media.[15] Congenital keratinizing cysts reported in humans and late recognition of slow-growing cysts may represent congenital keratinizing cysts in young to middle-aged dogs.[15] Clinical presentation can vary significantly and depends on the rapidity of growth and extent of damage. Although all are considered benign, some have a more aggressive biologic behavior. All can initiate resorption and remodeling of adjacent bone subsequent to chronic pressure. In all dogs, head shaking and pawing at the ear are common clinical signs, whereas otorrhea, discomfort at opening of the mouth, neurologic abnormalities including head tilt, facial paralysis, ataxia, and dysphagia are less common[16] and typically associated with more advanced disease. Rarely, these cysts may initially present as a nasopharyngeal mass.[17] The clinical history typically includes chronic, recurrent otitis externa/media, which is unresponsive or refractory to topical or systemic treatment. On otoscopy, presence of a pearly white growth, or white-to-yellow scales within the middle ear cavity, is highly suggestive.[16]

Computed tomography may be particularly useful in confirming this diagnosis. In a study of 11 dogs with aural keratinizing cysts, common computed tomography findings included osteoproliferation (81.8%); osteolysis (72.7%); or osteosclerosis (45.4%) of the tympanic bulla. Although these can also be found in otitis media and neoplastic diseases, expansion of the bulla (90.9%) and lack of distinct contrast enhancement (a particular feature of neoplasia) is considered highly supportive of a diagnosis of an aural keratinizing cyst.[18]

Treatment consists of surgical removal by lateral or ventral bulla osteotomy, with or without ear canal ablation. Recurrence is frequent and associated with failure to remove all of the keratinizing epithelium, or failure to control associated otitis externa/media. Recurrence is associated with advanced disease on initial presentation for surgery as indicated by inability to open the jaw, neurologic disease, or evidence of boney lysis on imaging.[15]

Cholesterol Granulomas

Cholesterol granulomas are benign, granulomatous lesions typified by the presence of abundant cholesterol aggregates (cholesterol clefts) within a granulomatous inflammatory matrix. They are uncommonly reported in the middle ear of dogs primarily in association with chronic otitis media, and when advanced, can cause osteitis and erosion of bone.[19] Risk factors for development include hemorrhage, obstruction of ventilation, or obstruction of normal drainage at a site of inflammation. They have been reported as a complication of total ear canal ablation and lateral ventral bulla osteotomy,[20] and as spontaneous findings. The primary differential diagnosis for cholesterol granulomas is aural keratinizing cysts, which can present similarly, but typically cause more local boney destruction and more severe clinical signs. Not surprisingly, given their common association with chronic inflammation, in a study of 11 dogs with middle ear aural keratinizing cysts, 4 had concurrent cholesterol granulomas.[18]

Treatment is based on surgical excision of the inflammatory mass, which in the early stages may have the appearance of regional mucosal thickening, but when advanced may appear as a yellow, round to irregular, variably friable mass within the tympanic cavity.[19]

Cysts

Feline ceruminous cystomatosis

Ceruminous cystomatosis is an uncommon, nonneoplastic disorder characterized by multiple, punctate, usually pigmented nodules or vesicles within the external ear canal and inner pinna. The cause is unknown. A frequent association with chronic otitis externa has been reported; however, a congenital or degenerative cause is also considered. Affected animals are typically late to middle aged, but the condition has been reported in cats younger than 1 year old. A slight male predominance, and increased frequently in Abyssinian and Persian cats has been reported.[21] Diagnosis is typically not difficult given the relatively unique presentation, although the pigmented masses may be mistaken clinically for a melanotic or vascular neoplasm.

Follicular cysts

Follicular cysts are nonneoplastic dilations of hair follicles. Typically, they are benign entities and excision is curative. One report of multiple follicular cysts within the external ear canal presented as chronic otitis externa, para-auricular swelling, fistulation, and an extensive soft tissue mass effect extending from the external ear canal into the tympanic bulla.[5]

Noninfectious Cutaneous Granulomatous Lesions

In dogs and cats, numerous granulomatous skin lesions may involve the pinna, most presenting as discreet papules, nodules, or plaques that may be localized or generalized. Although infectious agents can typically be identified on routine histopathology, a broad array of "sterile" lesions categorizes those cases where infectious agents are not readily identified. With the advancement of molecular techniques including polymerase chain reaction, immunohistochemistry, and in situ hybridization, many infectious agents are now being identified in lesions previously considered "sterile." Noninfectious, granulomatous lesions include sterile granuloma and pyogranuloma syndrome, cutaneous xanthoma, canine sarcoidosis, and foreign body reactions.

Sterile granuloma and pyogranuloma syndrome
Sterile granuloma and pyogranuloma syndrome is a heterogenous group of nodular skin lesions with similar histologic features that are uncommon in dogs and rare in cats. Lesions are typically multiple, firm, well-demarcated, variably sized dermal plaques or nodules that typically affect the head, particularly muzzle, pinnae, and periorbital regions.[22] In the cat, the muzzle is more commonly affected, but lesions also occur on the pinnae, extremities, and paw pads. Additional diagnostics should be used to rule out the fastidious, and difficult to culture mycobacteria of the canine leproid granuloma and the protozoan, *Leishmania* spp, in these lesions.

Cutaneous xanthoma
Cutaneous xanthomas typically present as bilaterally symmetric, preauricular multifocal to coalescing, white-yellow plaques or nodules in the cat, and very rarely the dog, and are considered a manifestation of dyslipoproteinemia. Lipid deposits occur in a variety of tissues, including the skin of the pinna, and may be quite extensive in severe cases.[22]

Other Nonneoplastic Mass Effects of the Ear

Aural hematomas
Aural hematomas are fluid-filled swellings that typically develop on the concave surface of the pinna in dogs and cats. The cause is not clear; however, it is commonly accepted that they develop secondary to trauma and rupture of blood vessels within the pinnae. Affected animals typically present with a history that includes persistent head shaking or scratching at the ears, most commonly secondary to otitis externa. Diagnosis is typically straightforward and treatment is surgical drainage and close apposition of the skin to the auricular cartilage.

Auricular chondritis and chondrosis (relapsing polychondritis)
Auricular chondritis/chondrosis is presumptively an autoimmune, rare disorder of young to middle-aged cats (reported in one dog) causing a markedly swollen, curled, and painful pinna with intense erythema that although initially unilateral usually progresses to involve both pinnae. Animals typically present systemically ill, and diagnosis is based on hematologic findings of neutrophilia, lymphocytosis, and hyperglobulinemia, paired with typical histopathologic findings.[23] Auricular chondritis resembles relapsing polychondritis in humans, a rare condition affecting cartilage in many sites and associated with ocular and cardiovascular disease. Lesions are typically limited to the pinna in cats; however, cases have described extra-auricular chondritis and ocular and cardiovascular lesions.[24,25] Treatment options include immunosuppressive therapy, dapsone, and pinnectomy. Recurrent disease (relapsing) has not been reported in cats.[24]

Idiopathic benign lichenoid keratosis
Idiopathic benign lichenoid keratosis is a rare condition seen in dogs of any age that typically presents as multiple, well circumscribed, wart-like papules or hyperkeratotic plaques. Lesions are typically unilateral and localized to the concave surface of the pinna.[26] Surgical excision is curative.

Lichenoid-psoriasiform dermatosis of springer spaniels
The appearance of lichenoid-psoriasiform dermatosis lesions is similar to that of idiopathic benign lichenoid keratosis; however, this entity occurs only in young springer spaniels and bilateral pinnal involvement is expected. Lesions may also occur on other areas of the body.[26]

Eosinophilic dermatitis
Nodular eosinophilic dermatitides are common occurrences in the cat. Two distinct forms, the feline eosinophilic plaque and feline eosinophilic granuloma, commonly involve the head. Eosinophilic dermatitis is less frequently described in the dog, and is typified by eosinophilic granulomas, typically within the oral cavity. Eosinophilic granulomas are rarely reported as cutaneous entities, but have been reported on the pinna and as obstructive masses within the ear canal of dogs, presenting as single, but occasionally multiple, polypoid, white, granular masses.[27]

Craniomandibular osteopathy
Craniomandibular osteopathy is a genetic disorder particularly common to many terrier breeds that results in irregular thickening of the bones of the head, and in particular the tympanic bullae. In radiographic evaluations, this disease may present as irregular thickening and a mass-like effect within the tympanic bulla.[28]

BENIGN NEOPLASTIC DISEASES
Papilloma

Exophytic cutaneous papillomas present as single or multiple papillated sessile or pedunculated masses, typically less than 1 cm in diameter, most commonly occurring on the face, ears, and extremities of young dogs (<2 years old). These papillomas are associated with a papilloma virus distinct from canine oral papillomavirus and may spontaneously regress over a period of weeks to months.[29] Malignant transformation has rarely been reported. In older animals, papillomas typically are solitary and not associated with a viral origin. Surgical excision or cryosurgery is usually curative in those cases where spontaneous regression does not occur. There is a single report of a polypoid squamous papilloma originating from the external ear canal and extending into the middle ear. No significant boney changes were reported within the middle ear.[30]

Canine Cutaneous Histiocytoma

Canine cutaneous histiocytomas are benign neoplasms of Langerhans (histiocytic) cell origin,[31] with preferential location to the head and pinna. Tumors most frequently occur in young dogs (<4 years old) but occur in dogs of all ages. Masses generally arise as a single, ulcerated "button" lesion (**Fig. 1**) and typically resolve within several months. Rarely, multiple neoplasms may occur (persistent and recurrent cutaneous histiocytomas) with lymph node involvement (Langerhans cell histiocytosis); however, spontaneous resolution is still expected.[32] Diagnosis is generally straightforward and can be made cytologically or histologically. In rare instances where multiple or nonregressing nodules may clinically mimic a more malignant histiocytic process, immunohistochemical staining with anti–E-cadherin antibodies is available on formalin-fixed

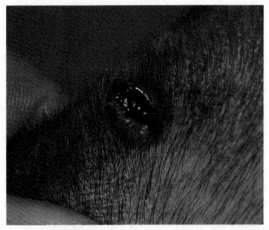

Fig. 1. Pinnal margin, dog. This discretely raised, red, alopecic, cutaneous neoplasm is the typical "button tumor" classic for canine cutaneous histiocytoma. This neoplasm has been centrally incised, but often these have crusted and ulcerated surfaces. (*Courtesy of* Dr L.K. Cole, College of Veterinary Medicine, Ohio State University, Columbus, OH.)

paraffin sections and is effective for definitively identifying canine cutaneous histiocytomas from their more malignant counterparts and other leukocytic neoplasms.[33] Treatment is generally unnecessary, but may be considered in older patients or when the lesion does not spontaneously regress.

Plasmacytoma

Plasma cell tumors are common, benign neoplasms in dogs and cats with particular predilection to the feet, lips, and ear canal (**Fig. 2**).[34] These neoplasms typically arise

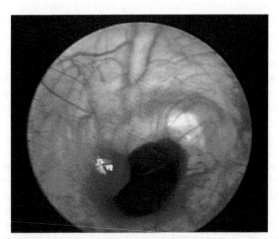

Fig. 2. Plasmacytoma, external ear canal (cleaned and depilated), dog. A small, discreet, raised mass in the ear canal is most typical for a plasmacytoma; however, cytologic or histopathologic evaluation is required to definitively differentiate this from other neoplasms that may, at least initially, appear similar. (*Courtesy of* Dr L.K. Cole, College of Veterinary Medicine, Ohio State University, Columbus, OH.)

as single and occasionally multiple well-demarcated, rapidly growing masses. Diagnosis is straightforward through cytologic and histopathologic examination. Complete excision is curative.

Other Benign Neoplasia

Basal cell tumors, rhabdomyomas (cat), fibromas, hemangiomas, mast cell tumors, sebaceous adenomas, and melanocytomas have all been reported on the pinna of dogs and cats.[9] In all cases, complete surgical resection is effective to control local disease.

Other rare, benign neoplasms reported in cats include two papillary adenomas of the middle ear[30] and a single, mature, para-auricular teratoma.[35]

MALIGNANT NEOPLASTIC DISEASES

Malignant neoplastic diseases are most commonly diagnosed in the external ear canal of dogs and cats. Ceruminous gland adenocarcinoma, squamous cell carcinoma (SCC), and carcinoma of undetermined origin are most frequently diagnosed. In a large study of neoplasms of the external ear canal, median survival time of dogs with malignant aural neoplasia was greater than 58 months, and only 11.7 months in cats.[36] This overall shorter survival time correlates with the observation that aural tumors tend to be more biologically aggressive in cats,[1] and further that most aural neoplasms are malignant in cats (85%) compared with dogs (60%). Negative prognostic indicators in dogs and cats include a diagnosis of SCC, carcinoma of undetermined origin, or clinical signs of neurologic disease. Further negative prognostic indicators include extensive local infiltration of the tumor in dogs and evidence of lymphatic or vascular invasion in cats.[36] In dogs, local invasion is common, but distant metastasis of malignant auricular neoplasms is uncommon. Radiographic evidence of thoracic metastasis was found in 3 (8.6%) of 35 dogs examined in one study of ear canal tumors.[36] Radiographic evidence of thoracic metastasis was not detected in 32 cats with malignant auricular tumors in the same study; however, 5 (8.9%) of 56 cats had cytologic evidence of lymph node involvement.

Neoplasia within the middle and internal ear is much less common and is typically the result of direct extension of a neoplasm from a more lateral compartment. Middle ear cavity neoplasia constitutes only 2% to 6% of referrals for aural surgery in the dog.[30] SCC is the most common neoplasm to arise from the middle ear, although its occurrence is rare in dogs and cats. Other rarely reported neoplasms thought to arise primarily within the middle ear of the dog include an adenoma of the eustachian tube, two paragangliomas, and a fibromyxoma.[9] Scattered reports of primary middle ear neoplasia in cats include SCC, most frequently, and rare reports of carcinoma of undetermined origin, lymphoma, and fibrosarcoma.[9]

Although the internal ear is composed of mesenchymal, epithelial, and neural cell types, any of which may undergo neoplastic transformation, neoplasia definitely determined to be of internal ear origin has not been reported in domestic animals. Patients presenting with clinical signs attributable to internal ear disease are more likely to be affected with bacterial otitis interna, trauma, or idiopathic peripheral vestibular disease.

Any neoplasia involving the temporal bone may produce signs of internal ear disease, primarily peripheral vestibular signs (head tilt, pathologic nystagmus), and variable degrees of Horner syndrome or other cranial nerve deficits.[37] Documented cases in the veterinary literature include fibrosarcoma; osteosarcoma; chondrosarcoma;

SCC; lymphoma; and adnexal (ceruminous and sebaceous) gland adenocarcinoma.[38] Limited reports with radiographic confirmation of petrous temporal bone involvement include two geriatric cats diagnosed with a papillary adenocarcinoma of undetermined origin originating in the middle ear,[39] a fibrosarcoma of middle ear origin invading the petrous portion of the temple bone, multiple middle ear SCCs, and a single report of a poorly differentiated carcinoma of nasopharyngeal origin with invasion into the internal ear.[40] In all tumors of the middle and internal ear, extension of the associated otitis and less often the neoplasm into the internal ear and cranium are associated with progressive neurologic dysfunction and rapid clinical deterioration.[37]

In contrast to humans, where metastasis to the auricular structures is documented to arise with some regularity from primary breast, lung, kidney, stomach, prostate, and laryngeal cancers,[41] metastasis to the ear is an uncommon, or poorly documented event in veterinary oncology.

Squamous Cell Carcinoma

SCC is a common, cutaneous tumor in dogs and cats, the cause of which may vary depending on primary location. Regardless of location, SCCs are locally invasive, highly malignant neoplasms that arise from squamous epithelial cells. SCCs are typically proliferative, poorly demarcated, and ulcerated, with frequent hemorrhage secondary to trauma. Treatment in early cases is surgical excision. Although these neoplasms are late to metastasize, recurrence is common. Adjunctive therapy for incompletely excised or recurrent neoplasms include cryosurgery, photodynamic, laser, or radiation therapy, and systemic or intralesional chemotherapy.[9]

SCC of the Auricle
SCCs of the ear are most commonly reported on the dorsal ear tips and lightly haired preauricular areas of cats, associated with chronic UV exposure. White cats have a 13.4 times greater risk of developing UV-associated lesions than colored cats.[42] Diagnosis can sometimes be delayed because these neoplasms typically present as bilateral lesions that progress from sites of hyperemia to thickened, crusty, ulcerated masses that may initially be mistaken for inflammatory lesions. Although diagnosis is typically straightforward on histopathologic evaluation, depending on the site and timing of the biopsy, histopathologic evaluation may reflect any stage of a continuum from actinic dermatosis to carcinoma in situ to locally invasive and aggressive SCC. In the dog, pinnal SCC is less commonly reported than the cat, but has similar etiologic ties to chronic UV exposure.[43]

SCC of the External Ear Canal and Middle Ear
SCC of the external ear canal is more commonly reported in dogs, but occurs in dogs and cats. In SCC of the external ear canal, chronic otitis externa is the most common associated clinical condition. Damaged skin and continuous exposure to carcinogenic ceruminous discharge from the ear are considered predisposing factors in development of SCC in this location.[43] Animals may present with a history of chronic otitis externa with recent onset of otorrhagia. Infrequent reports of SCC carcinoma arising either within the middle ear or extending from the external acoustic meatus has been reported in both species, and is considered the most common (although rare) neoplasm of the canine and feline middle ear.[1] In addition to typical signs of middle ear disease, clinical signs of SCC within the middle ear of dogs commonly include pain on opening the mouth resulting from advanced local tissue destruction of the surrounding bony structures.

Adnexal Neoplasms

Neoplastic transformation of adnexal structures is the most common neoplasia of the external ear canal in dogs and cats. These masses most commonly occur in middle-aged to older animals. Chronic local inflammation, ceruminous gland hyperplasia, and increased exposure to cerumen (increased production and decreased rate of removal) are considered predisposing factors for development.[1] Animals typically present with signs indistinguishable from otitis externa/media and concurrent otitis externa/media is a typical finding.

Ceruminous Gland Adenoma and Adenocarcinoma

Ceruminous glands are modified apocrine sweat glands. Neoplastic transformation of these glands is the most common neoplasm found in the external ear canal. Tumors typically originate within the external ear canal and are less common than tumors originating within the inner surface of the proximal pinna. Although ceruminous gland adenomas have historically been considered more common than carcinomas in the dog, carcinomas may be more frequent in dogs and cats.[44] Ceruminous gland adenomas typically appear as multiple, small, pedunculated, pigmented masses that are variably irregular and firm, whereas adenocarcinomas are typically irregularly raised to plaquelike, variably ulcerated, and locally invasive. Up to 50% of tumors metastasize to regional lymph nodes, lungs, and viscera,[45] although this high rate of metastasis is not consistently reported.[44] In a study of 124 ceruminous gland neoplasms, relative containment by the auricular cartilage is reported in most malignant tumors; however, extension to the middle ear and surrounding soft tissues of the parotid region[40] has been described. In a large study of ceruminous gland tumors, an almost invariable association between presence of this neoplasm and concurrent suppurative to pyogranulomatous inflammation[44] supports a causal relationship between chronic otitis externa and development of this neoplasm. Rarely, mixed ceruminous gland adenocarcinomas[44] and chondroid metaplasia at multiple metastatic foci[46] have been described.

Sebaceous Gland Adenoma and Adenocarcinoma

Reports of malignant sebaceous neoplasms are much less common than their ceruminous counterpart and may be attributed to fewer sebaceous glands subjected to chronic inflammation within the external ear canal. Biologic behavior is similar to ceruminous gland adenocarcinomas. In dogs, all sebaceous nodular diseases, nodular sebaceous hyperplasia, sebaceous adenomas, sebaceous epitheliomas (intermediate-grade malignancy), and sebaceous adenocarcinomas, occur most commonly on the head, with variable predilection for the pinna and dorsum,[11] and are not associated with chronic inflammatory otitis.

Vascular Neoplasms

Vascular tumors of the skin are uncommon, and in cats comprised 8 (3.3%) of 340 of all cutaneous neoplasms in one study.[47] In cats, the neoplasms are more commonly malignant, and hemangiosarcomas are typically localized to the head with greater than 50% occurring on the pinnae. Similar to SCC, hemangiosarcomas may be preferentially located on the ear tips of light-colored cats in association with chronic UV exposure.[47,48] Distant metastasis of cutaneous hemangiosarcoma has not been reported, but recurrence after excision is common.

In contrast to cats where malignant vascular tumors are more common, in the dog, benign cutaneous and subcutaneous hemangiomas are most frequent and occur anywhere on the body. As in cats, development of cutaneous hemangiosarcomas in the dog is associated with chronic UV exposure[49] at sites of lightly pigmented or minimally haired skin; however, there is no documented predilection for localization to the ear. Additionally, although uncommon, cutaneous hemangiosarcomas may represent metastatic foci of a primary visceral hemangiosarcoma, especially if present in an area less susceptible to chronic UV damage.

Feline Sarcoids and Feline Cutaneous Fibropapilloma

Feline sarcoids are neoplastic growths of fibroblasts associated with infection by a papillomavirus identified as feline sarcoid-associated papilloma virus. DNA sequencing of feline sarcoid-associated papilloma virus indicates this virus is most closely related to bovine papilloma virus-1, the induction agent of equine sarcoids.[50] Recent work indicates that feline sarcoid-associated papilloma virus can infect bovine skin, suggesting that cattle are the reservoir hosts of this papilloma virus, and that development of feline sarcoids could be the result of cross-species infection in a dead-end host.[51] Tumors are most commonly reported in rural, young (<1 year old) male cats with known exposure to cattle.[50]

Although the route of infection is not clearly identified, sarcoids occur most commonly on the head with the nares, lips, and pinnae most commonly affected. Given the propensity to localize to the head, marking behavior[52] and direct inoculation secondary to fighting, have been implicated as contributing factors. Less commonly, distal limbs, abdomen, and a single case within the external ear canal[50] have been described. Treatment is surgical excision. Although metastasis has not been reported, these neoplasms are highly infiltrative and local recurrence, with subsequent increased rate of regrowth, is common. Cryosurgery or radiation therapy may be effective in some cases.[52]

This entity should not be confused with canine sarcoidosis, a rare, idiopathic, nodular, skin disease of dogs characterized by multiple noncaseating, epitheloid granulomatous inflammatory nodules.[53] Canine sarcoidosis predominantly affects the trunk and head.

Cutaneous Lymphoma

Lymphoma is a common neoplastic disease in dogs and cats, and is the most common neoplasia in cats. Its occurrence as a primary cutaneous entity is uncommon, and comprises less than 2% of lymphoma in cats.[54] Cutaneous lymphoma occurs in two forms: epitheliotropic, with tissue tropism for the epidermis and adnexal epithelium; and nonepitheliotropic (dermal). Both forms are typically T cell in origin. Mucocutaneous involvement and epitheliotropic forms of the disease are more common in the dog.

Clinically, cutaneous, particularly epitheliotropic lymphoma, varies greatly in dogs and cats, but typically presents as scaly, alopecic patches and nonhealing ulcers or nodules without site predilection. Involvement of the ear is typically part of systemic disease. Cutaneous lymphoma may mimic eosinophilic plaques in cats, SCC, or any other ulcerated, inflammatory mass of the pinna (**Fig. 3**), and histopathology is required to definitively differentiate these neoplasms from each other and from reactive lymphocytic dermatitis and cutaneous lymphocytosis.

Other Malignant Tumors

Other reported malignant neoplasms of the ear include anaplastic carcinomas, adenocarcinomas, basal cell carcinomas,[30,55] hemangiopericytoma,[55] sarcoma,[55] malignant melanoma, paraganglioma,[56] mast cell tumors,[10] and a leiomyosarcoma.[10]

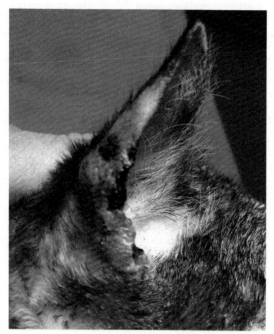

Fig. 3. Right pinna (clipped and cleaned), cat. Irregularly thickened to nodular, crusty, and ulcerative lesion of the lateral margin of the right pinna clinically suggestive of a squamous cell carcinoma. Cytologic evaluation of an aspirate revealed a monomorphic population of neoplastic lymphocytes, consistent with cutaneous lymphoma. Cutaneous lymphoma was also localized to an ulcerated lesion on the right rear foot. (*Courtesy of* Dr R. Brown, South Carolina Veterinary Specialists, Columbia, SC.)

SUMMARY

In patients presenting with clinical signs localized to the ear, most cases can be attributed to a nonneoplastic disease processes, such as otitis externa/media, trauma, or idiopathic peripheral vestibular disease. It is only in a small portion of patients where the typical spectrum of clinical signs point to neoplastic or other space-occupying, obstructive disorders. Clinical histories for most entities are typically nonspecific and frequently include chronic otitis externa/media/interna that is recurrent or refractory to systemic and topical treatments. Although further localization can often be achieved based on the particular spectrum of clinical signs, advanced disease often involves multiple components of the auricular structure, which may complicate the diagnostic picture. Furthermore, diagnosis may be made difficult by virtue of limited physical access to much of the auricular structures. As such, advanced imaging, cytology (fine-needle aspiration, scrape preparations), and histopathology are essential tools and should be used early on in the diagnostic process.

REFERENCES

1. Rogers KS. Tumors of the ear canal. Vet Clin North Am Small Anim Pract 1988;18: 859–68.
2. Malik R, Love DN, Wigney DI, et al. Mycobacterial nodular granulomas affecting the subcutis and skin of dogs (canine leproid granuloma syndrome). Aust Vet J 1998;76:403–7, 398.

3. Trainor KE, Porter BF, Logan KS, et al. Eight cases of feline cutaneous leishmaniasis in Texas. Vet Pathol 2010;47:1076–81.
4. White PD. Chronic proliferative otitis: now what, in small animal and exotics. North American Veterinary Conference. Orlando, FL, USA, January 8–12, 2005. 2005;827–9.
5. Gatineau M, Lussier B, Alexander K. Multiple follicular cysts of the ear canal in a dog. J Am Anim Hosp Assoc 2010;46:107–14.
6. Pratschke KM. Inflammatory polyps of the middle ear in 5 dogs. Vet Surg 2003; 32:292–6.
7. Forster-van Hijfte MA, Groth AM, Emmerson TD. Expansile, inflammatory middle ear disease causing nasopharyngeal obstruction in a cat. J Feline Med Surg 2011;13:451–3.
8. Anderson DM, Robinson RK, White RA. Management of inflammatory polyps in 37 cats. Vet Rec 2000;147:684–7.
9. Fan TM, de Lorimier LP. Inflammatory polyps and aural neoplasia. Vet Clin North Am Small Anim Pract 2004;34:489–509.
10. Bacon NJ, Gilbert RL, Bostock DE, et al. Total ear canal ablation in the cat: indications, morbidity and long-term survival. J Small Anim Pract 2003;44:430–4.
11. Gross TL, Ihrke PJ, Walder EJ, et al. Sebaceous tumors. In: Skin diseases of the dog and cat: clinical and histopathologic diagnosis. Oxford (United Kingdom): Blackwell Publishing Company; 2005. p. 641–54.
12. Mauldin EA, Ness TA, Goldschmidt MH. Proliferative and necrotizing otitis externa in four cats. Vet Dermatol 2007;18:370–7.
13. Gross TL, Ihrke PJ, Walder EJ, et al. Necrotizing diseases of the epidermis. In: Skin disease of the dog and cat: clinical and histopathologic diagnosis. Oxford (United Kingdom): Blackwell Publishing Company; 2005. p. 79–80.
14. Videmont E, Pin D. Proliferative and necrotising otitis in a kitten: first demonstration of T-cell-mediated apoptosis. J Small Anim Pract 2010;51:599–603.
15. Hardie EM, Linder KE, Pease AP. Aural cholesteatoma in twenty dogs. Vet Surg 2008;37:763–70.
16. Greci V, Travetti O, Di Giancamillo M, et al. Middle ear cholesteatoma in 11 dogs. Can Vet J 2011;52:631–6.
17. Ellison GW, Donnell RL, Daniel GB. Nasopharyngeal epidermal cyst in a dog. J Am Vet Med Assoc 1995;207:1590–2.
18. Travetti O, Giudice C, Greci V, et al. Computed tomography features of middle ear cholesteatoma in dogs. Vet Radiol Ultrasound 2010;51:374–9.
19. Fliegner RA, Jubb KV, Lording PM. Cholesterol granuloma associated with otitis media and destruction of the tympanic bulla in a dog. Vet Pathol 2007;44:547–9.
20. Riedinger B, Albaric O, Gauthier O. Cholesterol granuloma as long-term complication of total ear canal ablation in a dog. J Small Anim Pract 2011;53:188–91.
21. Gross TL, Ihrke PJ, Walder EJ, et al. Sweat gland tumors. In: Skin diseases of the dog and cat: clinical and histopathologic diagnosis. Oxford (United Kingdom): Blackwell Publishing Company; 2005. p. 667–8.
22. Gross TL. Skin diseases of the dog and cat: clinical and histopathologic diagnosis. 2nd edition. Ames (IA): Blackwell Science; 2005.
23. Matousek JL. Diseases of the ear pinna. Vet Clin North Am Small Anim Pract 2004;34:511–40.
24. Gerber B, Crottaz M, von Tscharner C, et al. Feline relapsing polychondritis: two cases and a review of the literature. J Feline Med Surg 2002;4:189–94.
25. Baba T, Shimizu A, Ohmuro T, et al. Auricular chondritis associated with systemic joint and cartilage inflammation in a cat. J Vet Med Sci 2009;71:79–82.

26. Anderson WI, Scott DW, Luther PB. Idiopathic benign lichenoid keratosis on the pinna of the ear in four dogs. Cornell Vet 1989;79:179–84.
27. Poulet FM, Valentine BA, Scott DW. Focal proliferative eosinophilic dermatitis of the external ear canal in four dogs. Vet Pathol 1991;28:171–3.
28. Gawor JP. Case reports of four cases of craniomandibular osteopathy. European Journal of Companion Animal Practice 2004;14:209–13.
29. Gross TL, Ihrke PJ, Walder EJ, et al. Epidermal tumors. In: Skin diseases of the dog and cat: clinical and histopathologic diagnosis. Oxford (United Kingdom): Blackwell Publishing Company; 2005. p. 567–8.
30. Little CJ, Pearson GR, Lane JG. Neoplasia involving the middle ear cavity of dogs. Vet Rec 1989;124:54–7.
31. Moore PF, Schrenzel MD, Affolter VK, et al. Canine cutaneous histiocytoma is an epidermotropic Langerhans cell histiocytosis that expresses CD1 and specific beta 2-integrin molecules. Am J Pathol 1996;148:1699–708.
32. Gross TL, Ihrke PJ, Walder EJ, et al. Histiocytic tumors. In: Skin diseases of the dog and cat: clinical and histopathologic diagnosis. Oxford (United Kingdom): Blackwell Publishing Company; 2005. p. 840–5.
33. Fulmer AK, Mauldin GE. Canine histiocytic neoplasia: an overview. Can Vet J 2007;48:1041–3, 1046–50.
34. Lucke VM. Primary cutaneous plasmacytomas in the dog and cat. J Small Anim Pract 1987;28:49–55.
35. Van Goethem B, Bosmans T, Chiers K. Surgical resection of a mature teratoma on the head of a young cat. J Am Anim Hosp Assoc 2010;46:121–6.
36. London CA, Dubilzeig RR, Vail DM, et al. Evaluation of dogs and cats with tumors of the ear canal: 145 cases (1978-1992). J Am Vet Med Assoc 1996;208:1413–8.
37. Rossmeisl JH Jr. Vestibular disease in dogs and cats. Vet Clin North Am Small Anim Pract 2010;40:81–100.
38. LeCouteur RA. Feline vestibular diseases: new developments. J Feline Med Surg 2003;5:101–8.
39. Lucroy MD, Vernau KM, Samii VF, et al. Middle ear tumours with brainstem extension treated by ventral bulla osteotomy and craniectomy in two cats. Vet Comp Oncol 2004;2:234–42.
40. Holzworth J. Diseases of the cat: medicine & surgery. Philadelphia: Saunders; 1987.
41. Devaney KO, Boschman CR, Willard SC, et al. Tumours of the external ear and temporal bone. Lancet Oncol 2005;6:411–20.
42. Dorn CR, Taylor DO, Schneider R. Sunlight exposure and risk of developing cutaneous and oral squamous cell carcinomas in white cats. J Natl Cancer Inst 1971; 46:1073–8.
43. Miller WH Jr, Shanley KJ. Bilateral pinnal squamous cell carcinoma in a dog with chronic otitis externa. Vet Dermatol 1991;2:3.
44. Moisan PG, Watson GL. Ceruminous gland tumors in dogs and cats: a review of 124 cases. J Am Anim Hosp Assoc 1996;32:448–52.
45. Legendre AM, Krahwinkel DJ Jr. Feline ear tumors. J Am Anim Hosp Assoc 1981; 17:1035–7.
46. Romanucci M, Malatesta D, Marinelli A, et al. Aural carcinoma with chondroid metaplasia at metastatic sites in a dog. Vet Dermatol 2011;22:373–7.
47. Miller MA, Nelson SL, Turk JR, et al. Cutaneous neoplasia in 340 cats. Vet Pathol 1991;28:389–95.
48. Miller MA, Ramos JA, Kreeger JM. Cutaneous vascular neoplasia in 15 cats: clinical, morphologic, and immunohistochemical studies. Vet Pathol 1992;29:329–36.

49. Goldschmidt MH, Hendrick MJ. Tumors of the skin and soft tissues. In: Meuten DJ, editor. Tumors in domestic animals. 4th edition. Ames (IA): Iowa State University Press; 2002. p. 99–101.
50. Hanna PE, Dunn D. Cutaneous fibropapilloma in a cat (feline sarcoid). Can Vet J 2003;44:601–2.
51. Munday JS, Knight CG. Amplification of feline sarcoid-associated papillomavirus DNA sequences from bovine skin. Vet Dermatol 2010;21(4):341–4.
52. Gross TL, Affolter VK. Advances in skin oncology. Third world congress of veterinary dermatology. Edinburgh, Scotland. September 11–14, 1996. 1998;382–5.
53. Scott DW, Noxon JO. Sterile sarcoidal granulomatous skin disease. Canine Practice 1990;15:11–5, 18.
54. Fontaine J, Heimann M, Day MJ. Cutaneous epitheliotropic T-cell lymphoma in the cat: a review of the literature and five new cases. Vet Dermatol 2011;22:454–61.
55. van der Gaag I. The pathology of the external ear canal in dogs and cats. Vet Q 1986;8:307–17.
56. Cooley AJ, Fox LE, Duncan ID, et al. Malignant jugulotympanic paraganglioma in a dog. J Comp Pathol 1990;102:375–83.

Feline Deafness

David K. Ryugo, PhD[a],*, Marilyn Menotti-Raymond, PhD[b]

KEYWORDS

- Auditory system • Brain • Cochlea • Congenital deafness • Genes • Synapse

KEY POINTS

- Cats have among the best hearing of all mammals in that they are extremely sensitive to a broad range of frequencies. The rattle of the cat's food box or the hiss of a can opening should be sufficient to summon your cat no matter where it is in the house. Failure to call your cat this way is a sign that it is ill or losing its hearing.
- The ear is a highly complex structure that is delicately balanced in terms of its biochemistry, types of receptors, ion channels, mechanical properties, and cellular organization. Minor perturbations of any component of hearing can cause loss of function.
- Sensorineural deafness is usually caused by "flawed" genes that are inherited from one or both parents. Defects can appear as a disturbance in chemistry, failure of the receptive sensory elements, or impaired biomechanics. Hearing loss can also be acquired as a result of noise trauma from industrialized environment, viral infection, or blunt trauma. To date, it is not practical to intervene and attempt to correct these forms of deafness in cats.

INTRODUCTION

The ability to hear sound is one of the fundamental ways that organisms are able to perceive the external environment. It is speculated that hearing evolved as a distance sense, a function driven by a need for animals to detect potential danger, food, or mates that could not be seen because of darkness or dense foliage. Animals have the ability to sense perturbations in the air, and in vertebrates, the internal ear is a highly developed sensory structure that enables this function. Cats have especially keen hearing.[1] Their ability to hunt, avoid predators and oncoming motor vehicles, and interact with their owners depends on their hearing. Cats with hearing loss and/or deafness are vulnerable to danger.

For terrestrial vertebrates, sound is created by vibrations in air.[2] These vibrations may be characterized by frequency (cycles per second, Hz), which is correlated to

D.K.R. is supported by NHMRC grant #1009842, The Garnett Passe and Rodney Williams Memorial Foundation, NSW Office of Science and Medical Research, the Curran Foundation, and NIH/NIDCD grant DC004395; M.M.R. is supported with federal funds from the National Cancer Institute, National Institutes of Health, under contract HHSN26120080001E.
The authors have nothing to disclose.
[a] Hearing Research Program, Garvan Institute of Medical Research, 384 Victoria Street, Sydney, New South Wales 2010, Australia; [b] Laboratory of Genomic Diversity, Frederick National Laboratory for Cancer Research, National Cancer Institute, Frederick, MD 21702, USA
* Corresponding author.
E-mail address: d.ryugo@garvan.org.au

the sensation of pitch, the magnitude of the pressure of the vibrations (loudness), their timing (eg, onset, offset, duration, cadence), and the location. Two ears allow the extraction of important acoustic cues: the ear closer to the sound source will hear the sound sooner (interaural timing difference) and louder (interaural level difference) than the more distant ear. These binaural differences allow the brain to calculate sound location, and survival can depend on knowing if the sound comes from the right or the left. Sound arriving from the front has a different character than sound arriving from behind owing to interference by the external ear. This interference is called a head-related transfer function. The cat learns about the transfer functions so that it can also distinguish between sound in the front and back, an ability that is important to survival.

Sound is captured by the pinna, the external portion of the ear, and funneled through the ear canal to the tympanic membrane or eardrum (**Fig. 1**). The tympanic membrane is mechanically coupled to the 3 middle ear ossicles (the malleus, incus, and stapes), whose combined function is to deliver the vibrations to the fluid-filled internal ear with the same power as that delivered to the tympanic membrane. The vibrations in air become vibrations in fluid and are transmitted to the sensory hair cell receptors that reside in the organ of Corti. This mechanical signal is converted to neural signals and relayed to the brain by the cochlear (or auditory) branch of cranial nerve VIII (also known as the vestibulocochlear nerve). The brain receives and interprets these signals and the result is what we perceive as hearing.

- Mammalian hearing relies on 2 broad categories of function: mechanical and electrochemical.
- The mechanical component involves the capture of sound by the external ear and its transmission into the fluid-filled cochlea. The vibrations in the fluids mechanically stimulate different regions of the internal ear based on frequency, where these perturbations mechanically stimulate the cochlear hair cell bundle.
- The electrochemical component results from specialized cells that border the endolymphatic space and create a unique chemical environment. The endolymph has a positive potential ($\sim$80 mV) that drives K^+ into the cytoplasm of stimulated hair cells. Receptor cell responses are converted to action potentials in fibers of the cochlear nerve and conveyed to the brain. Malfunction of either of these auditory processing components results in hearing loss.
- Two types of hearing loss are identified and considered as separate entities.

"Conductive" hearing loss refers to problems of the peripheral auditory system, whereas "sensorineural" hearing loss refers to malfunction of the neuronal components of the auditory system.

- "Conductive" hearing loss results from external ear occlusion, tympanic membrane perforation, ossicular chain discontinuity or fixation, or middle ear infections. For cats, conductive hearing loss is often amenable to improvement with cleaning the external ear canal, antibiotics to clear middle ear infection, or surgical procedures to repair the tympanic membrane or ossicular function.
- "Sensorineural" hearing loss, on the other hand, can result from pathology anywhere along the auditory pathway, from the hair cell receptors to higher-order central auditory processing centers. Deafness owing to sensorineural hearing loss resembles a train wreck: it can result from many diverse causes but the outcome is always hearing loss.
- Sensorineural deafness can be classified into 2 broad classes: congenital deafness and acquired deafness.

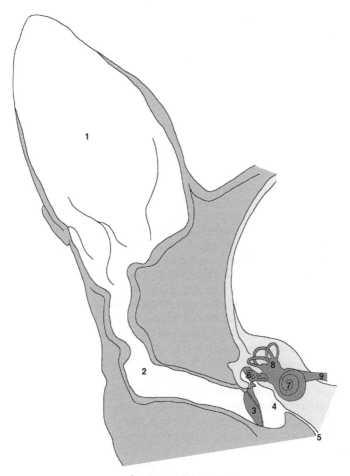

Anatomy of the cat ear

1. Pinna	6. Middle ear ossicles
2. External ear canal	malleus, incus, stapes
3. Tympanic membrane	7. Cochlea
4. Middle ear space	8. Vestibular apparatus
5. Eustacian tube	9. Auditory nerve

Fig. 1. Schematic drawing of the cat ear. The external ear consists of the pinna (1) and external ear canal (2) that conducts airborne sound to the tympanic membrane (3, ear drum). The tympanic membrane and 3 middle ear bones (6) occupy the middle ear space (4). These moving parts convert vibrations in air to vibrations in the inner ear (7). The middle ear space is confluent with the pharynx by way of the Eustachian tube (5). Behind the cochlea, the auditory component of the inner ear, lies the vestibular structures (8). The eighth cranial nerve, the auditory-vestibular nerve (9), conducts sensory information from the sense organ to the brain. (*Courtesy of* Catherine Connelly, Garvan Institute of Medical Research, Sydney, Australia.)

- Congenital deafness is a condition that exists at birth and often before birth, or that develops during the first month of life regardless of etiology. In humans, nearly half of the causes of deafness can be attributed to genetic abnormalities. One-third of these defects is accompanied by identified disorders in other systems, and is considered "syndromic" deafness. The remaining two-thirds, however, are isolated to hearing loss and considered "nonsyndromic."

- Acquired deafness refers to a loss of hearing that is not present at birth but develops during the animal's lifetime. The causes of acquired hearing loss can be illness (eg, meningitis), head trauma, ototoxic drugs, and exposure to loud noise. In industrialized society, cats exhibit a significant amount of "normal pathology" that is assumed to arise from street noise.[1]

GENETICS OF DEAFNESS

Considerable progress has been made in identifying the genes and genetic loci associated with mammalian deafness. The list of genes is more than 100 and an updated database of the nonsyndromic deafness genes and loci is maintained at the Hereditary Hearing Loss Homepage (http://hereditaryhearingloss.org). With the identification of hereditary deafness genes and the proteins they encode, molecular elements of basic hearing mechanisms emerge. As the function of these identified molecular elements continue to be unraveled, we can begin to understand the remarkable complexity of hearing. Multiple genes interact and express themselves at multiple loci such that rarely is a single gene responsible for the normal functioning of any system. The goal of this article was to summarize the function of some of the proteins implicated in hearing and genetic deafness while using the deaf white cat as the model (**Fig. 2**). The white cat is a good model for study because it has good low-frequency hearing like humans, and when deaf, its deafness is naturally occurring, has a genetic basis, and exhibits variable expression.

The deaf white cat has long held a fascination to humans, attracting the attention of Charles Darwin, among others.[3,4] The product of a single autosomal dominant locus, *White (W)*, demonstrates pleiotropic effects, including a white coat, blue iris, and deafness, all 3 of which can be attributed to an absence or abnormality of melanocytes. The correlation between white coat color, blue irises, and deafness is, however, imperfect. Thus, white cats exhibit a uniform white coat, although they can be born with a colored spot that fades with age, and they may be either unilaterally or bilaterally deaf, demonstrating varying degrees of severity, from mild to profound. Additionally, their irises are often blue because of the absence of melanin, and the likelihood of deafness has been calculated at 80% with the frequency of blue irises.[5,6]

The white, deaf phenotype has been reported in multiple species, including the mouse, dog, mink, horse, rat, Syrian hamster, alpaca, and human.[7–19] Type 2 Waardenburg syndrome most closely describes the phenotype in humans with distinctive

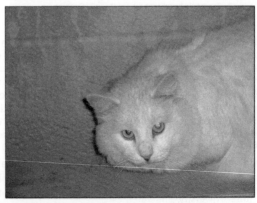

Fig. 2. A congenitally deaf white cat. Note the heterochromia of the irides. This particular cat is healthy with no balance deficiencies; only deafness. (*Courtesy of* Dr David K. Ryugo, Garvan Institute of Medical Research, Sydney, Australia.)

hypopigmentation of skin and hair and congenital cochleosaccule dysplasia that resembles the Scheibe deformity. Investigation of the genetic basis for distinctive coat color phenotypes represent some of the earliest mapped and characterized genetic mutations.[20] Early in embryogenesis, melanoblasts, or pigment precursor cells, migrate from the neural crest to the skin, regions of the eye, and the internal ear. Mutations affecting any step in this pathway, be it proliferation, survival, migration, or distribution of melanoblasts is often manifested as coat color variation. Genes identified in these early events of pigmentation, many of which were characterized in the mouse white-spotting mutants, include Pax3, Mitf, Slug, Ednrb, Edn3, Sox10 and Kit.[21–30]

In spite of the long-standing interest in coat color and deafness, only recently has the role of melanocytes in hearing been studied. In the internal ear, melanocytes are largely observed in the stria vascularis, the vascularized epithelium responsible for secreting high levels of K^+ into the endolymph, which establishes the endocochlear potential (EP).[31] The +80 mV EP is crucial for the normal function of the auditory receptor cells. Melanocytes are the only cell type in the stria vascularis to express the potassium channel protein, KCNJ10 (Kir4.1), providing the structural basis for the rate-limiting step that establishes the EP.[32] Knockouts of the Kcnj10 gene in mice eliminate the EP and reduce endolymph potassium concentration, with resultant deafness.[32]

The incomplete penetrance for iris color and deafness has made it challenging to interpret an individual's genetic condition by classic linkage approaches, because those who possess the particular gene will not necessarily exhibit features of the gene.[33] Reduced penetrance is thought to result from a combination of genetic, environmental, and lifestyle factors, many of which are not known. Our approach to this dilemma is to perform linkage analysis for White in a pedigree segregating for white coat color. Information on the mutational mechanism can be applied to the segregation of deafness in an extended pedigree to examine features associated with the incomplete penetrance for deafness (ie, the impact of homozygosity vs heterozygosity for the mutation on phenotype.) A pedigree segregating for White has been generated and a candidate gene approach is used by genotyping short tandem repeat loci (STRs), tightly linked to the strong candidate genes Pax3, Mitf, Slug, Ednrb, Edn3, Sox10, and Kit, previously noted as causative of hypopigmentation and deafness in other mammalian species.[21–30]

If significant linkage is not detected to a candidate gene, a whole genome scan will be performed using the newly available cat SNP chip.[34] The identified mutation will then be characterized in this extended colony and in a population genetic survey of cats (283 of registered breed, 19 mixed breed), including pigmented individuals and 34 unrelated Dominant White individuals to examine the correlation between the characterized mutation with white coat color and/or deafness.[35]

- White cats are neither necessarily deaf nor blue-eyed.
- Examination of a large white deaf colony revealed a correlation between the likelihood that an individual will be deaf and/or blue-eyed based on their genotype (homozygous or heterozygous) at W inferred from designed breeding studies.[36] This correlation does not mean that the relationship is causal.

A potential explanation to the reduced penetrance at the feline W locus has been suggested. Melanocytes can be subdivided into cutaneous and noncutaneous lineages that respond differently to KIT signaling during development.[37] Cutaneous or "classical" murine melanocytes that "color" skin and hair are highly sensitive to KIT signaling, whereas melanocytes that populate the internal ear and portions of the eye (iris and choroid) are more effectively stimulated by endothelin 3 (EDN3) or hepatocyte growth factor (HGF).[37]

KIT has recently been implicated in 2 hypopigmentation phenotypes in the cat: White Spotting (*S*), in which significant linkage has been reported to *KIT*,[38] and the glove gene.[39] The perceived lack of penetrance at *W* for deafness could be explained if *KIT* is identified as the feline *White* locus.[37] In individuals heterozygous for the mutation, some melanocytes could survive migration to the internal ear and iris, as they are less sensitive to a decrease in KIT signaling, as opposed to melanocytes destined to pigment hair, which are highly sensitive to KIT signaling. The completion of linkage analysis may provide the answer to this question of penetrance.

COCHLEAR ANATOMY AND PHYSIOLOGY

Understanding mechanisms of deafness begins with a basic knowledge of the normal anatomy and physiology of the auditory pathway. Because the auditory system is complicated, with many working parts, there are innumerable potential sources and locations where problems could arise. The first part of this review highlights structural and functional features of the peripheral and central auditory system. This background provides a context with which to review the pathophysiology of hereditary and acquired deafness.

The cochlea is a spiraled bony tube housing 3 fluid-filled chambers that spiral along its length (**Fig. 3**). Highly specialized cells within the cochlea regulate the ionic composition of these chambers. One chamber is folded back at the apex to form 2 outer chambers (scala tympani and scala vestibuli) that sandwich a middle chamber (scala media). These outer chambers are confluent at the apex and contain perilymph, a filtrate of cerebrospinal fluid of similar composition to extracellular fluid (eg, high sodium, low potassium). The middle chamber contains endolymph, a high-potassium, low-sodium fluid of similar composition to intracellular fluid. The outer wall of scala media is partially lined by the stria vascularis (see **Fig. 3**). The stria is a vascularized, multilayered epithelial structure formed by 3 different cell types: marginal, intermediate, and basal cells (**Fig. 4**). A superficial layer of marginal cells borders the endolymph. Pale-staining basal cells are linked to each other, to intermediate cells, and to fibrocytes of the spiral ligament by gap junctions. This network provides cytoplasmic confluence that allows the free diffusion of K^+ toward the marginal cells. Intermediate cells are marked by the presence of melanosomes and by deep infoldings of the plasma membrane that are matched by those of the overlying marginal cells. The resulting dense, labyrinthine membrane system of narrow compartments is filled with mitochondria and surround the penetrating capillaries that course longitudinally along the epithelium. The elaborate infoldings of membrane greatly amplify the cell surface so as to transfer K^+ into marginal cells for secretion into the endolymph.[40,41]

As a result of the differences in ionic composition between the compartments, the potential difference between endolymph and perilymph is about +80 mV. This positive potential is the largest found in the body. Because the intracellular resting potential of hair cell receptors is approximately −70 mV, the potential difference across the hair cell apex is a remarkable 150 mV. This large potential difference represents a tremendous ionic force and serves as the engine driving the mechanoelectrical transduction process of the hair cell.[42] Membrane specializations that feature gap junctions allow free passage of K^+ ions through fibrocytes and basal cells and into intermediate cells. K^+ channels and pumps transfer K^+ from intermediate cells into the intrastrial fluid and then it gets concentrated in the marginal cells. K^+ is driven into the endolymph down the K^+ concentration gradient established in the marginal cells. The cycling of K^+ through the receptor cells and back into the endolymph is key to normal cochlear function.

- Gap junctions are channels that allow rapid transport of ions and small molecules between cells. In the stria vascularis, the ion is potassium (K^+).

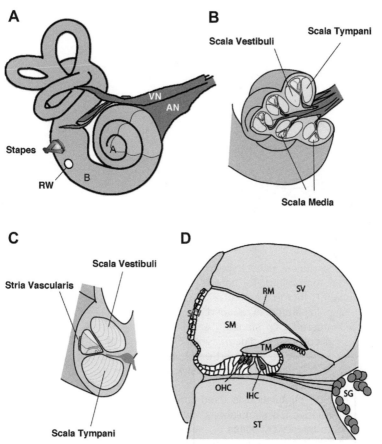

Fig. 3. Anatomy of the inner ear. (*A*) View of right hearing and balance apparatus. The cochlea is the coiled structure on the right and the semicircular canals of the vestibular system are on the left. For the cochlea, "A" indicates the apex (low frequencies) and "B" indicates the base (high frequencies). The stapes, a middle ear bone, inserts into the vestibule of the inner ear; the round window (RW) is covered by a membrane that relieves the pressure when the stapes "pistons" into the ear. The auditory (AN) and vestibular (VN) nerves bundle together to form the eighth cranial nerve. (*B*) A section of the otic capsule has been cut away (indicated in *A*) to reveal the 3 chambers of the labyrinth. The sensory organ resides in the scala media (*yellow*). (*C*) A rotated view of the cut end of a cochlear turn showing the 3 chambers, with the scala media (*yellow*) and the stria vascularis. (*D*) Enlarged diagram showing a cross-section through the scala media, emphasizing the organ of Corti and the hair cell receptors. IHC, inner hair cell; OHC, outer hair cells; RM, Reissner membrane; SG, spiral ganglion; SM, scala media; ST, scala tympani; StV, stria vascularis; SV, scala vestibuli; TM, tectorial membrane. (*Adapted from* Eisen MD, Ryugo DK. Hearing molecules: contributions from genetic deafness. Cell Mol Life Sci 2007;64(5):566–80; with permission.)

- Connexins are transmembrane proteins that form gap junction channels. Four different connexin molecules have been identified in the cochlea, including connexin 26, 30, 31, and 43.[43]
- Mutations that affect internal ear connexins result in hearing impairment and deafness.
- Mutations that affect K^+ transport result in hearing impairment and deafness.

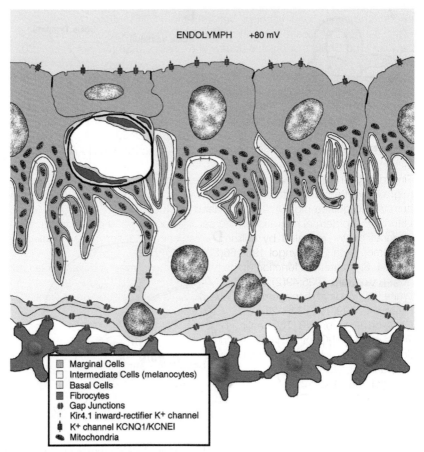

Fig. 4. Schematic drawing of the stria vascularis. Movement of K$^+$ ions through the gap junctions and then into the endolymph by way of ion pumps is crucial. This structure is the part of the inner ear that provides the special chemical environment that allows the system to function. (*Courtesy of* Dr David K. Ryugo, Garvan Institute of Medical Research, Sydney, Australia.)

Properties of the Cochlea

Sound vibrations are eventually delivered to the stapes, whose footplate serves as a kind of piston and imparts vibrations to the fluids of the scala vestibuli. Specializations within the cochlea decompose the mechanical stimulus of sound into its frequency components. The basilar membrane is a fibrous sheet stretched across the floor of scala media. Its width and thickness vary systematically from the base to the apex of the cochlea in that there is a continuous elasticity gradient from one end to the other. The base is narrow and thick, whereas the apex is wide and thin. This structure functions like a frequency analyzer where it resonates to high frequencies at the base and to progressively lower frequencies along toward the apex.

- The organ of Corti is the sensory organ for hearing.
- It is a multisensory structure that consists of the following:
  - Basilar membrane
  - Support cells

- ○ Inner hair cells that are the primary sensory receptor
- ○ Outer hair cells that modify the activity of the inner hair cells
- ○ The tectorial membrane

The organ of Corti rests on top of the basilar membrane (**Fig. 5**). Inner hair cells synapse onto afferent endings of the myelinated cochlear nerve fibers and are primarily responsible for conveying sensory information to the brain. In contrast, outer hair cells synapse on a small number of unmyelinated cochlear nerve fibers and receive large efferent nerve endings. The outer hair cells also contain contractile machinery that responds to membrane voltage changes. The outer hair cell's function appears more involved with amplifying and manipulating the sound stimulus. Specialized supporting cells in the organ of Corti complement the hair cells and have a vital role in maintaining the integrity and function of the hair cells. A final component of the cochlea's functional apparatus is the tectorial membrane, a gelatinous ribbon of extracellular matrix attached medially and contacting the outer hair cell hair bundles.

Hair Cell Anatomy, Function, and Innervation

Hair cells are polarized in that a bundle of stereocilia protrude from one end of the cell, their apex, which are composed of actin filaments (see **Fig. 5**), whereas afferent innervation occurs only at the opposite end, the base. Interconnecting links from the tip of a shorter stereocilia to the shaft of a longer neighbor, called "tip links," attach to the mechanoelectric transduction channel.[44,45] Mechanical oscillations of the basilar

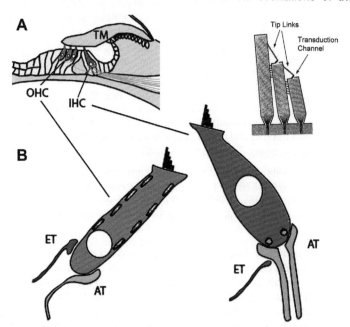

Fig. 5. Components of the organ of Corti. (*A*) The organ of Corti rests on the basilar membrane, and is composed of the sensory receptor cells (OHCs and IHCs), supporting cells (*yellow*), and the tectorial membrane (TM). (*B*) The hair cell receptors are innervated by afferent type I (*blue*) and type II (*green*) terminals, as well as by efferent (ET, *red*) terminals whose cell bodies reside in the brain stem. At the apical ends of the receptor cells are stereocilia that form part of the transduction apparatus with tip-links and channels (*upper right*). (*Adapted from* Eisen MD, Ryugo DK. Hearing molecules: contributions from genetic deafness. Cell Mol Life Sci 2007;64(5):566–80; with permission.)

membrane cause stereocilia within hair bundles to be displaced relative to each other. This displacement puts the tip links under tension and "pulls open" cation channels. Because of the high endocochlear potential, cations flow into the hair bundle and depolarize the hair cell membrane potential. Where the apical end of the cell transduces mechanical energy, the basal end releases neurotransmitter and activates afferent synapses.

The intracellular processes that respond to changes in membrane potential are distinctly different between the 2 types of auditory hair cells. Inner hair cells form afferent synapses where membrane voltage changes are converted to action potentials in myelinated cochlear nerve fibers; outer hair cells, however, contain electromotile elements within their cell membrane and generally serve as mechanical amplifiers of the sound stimuli for inner hair cells.[46]

The presynaptic machinery of inner hair cells is geared to generate graded release of neurotransmitter along their basolateral surface. Voltage-dependent Ca^{++} channels are localized with neurotransmitter release sites that open in response to membrane depolarization, which in turn results in the release of neurotransmitter. The amount of transmitter release is modulated by the magnitude of the membrane voltage change. Neurotransmitter diffuses across the synaptic cleft and binds to postsynaptic receptors on afferent dendrites of cochlear nerve fibers. This process begins the generation and propagation of action potentials along the afferent fibers.

Outer hair cells contain a contractile apparatus that responds to membrane voltage changes with contractions or elongations of the cell proper. This mechanical response appears to be conformational changes in cytoskeletal proteins of the plasma membrane wall that serve to modulate the oscillations transmitted to the inner hair cells' hair bundles. In addition to the electromotile apparatus within the outer hair cell, a system of efferent auditory feedback innervates the hair cells. Both systems work in concert to tune and amplify the sound source.[46]

The Spiral Ganglion

Spiral ganglion cells reside in Rosenthal's canal of the cochlea (**Fig. 6**). Their peripheral processes innervate the hair cell receptors, and their central processes conduct auditory information to the brain. Two types of ganglion cells have been described.[47,48]

- Type I ganglion cells are large (20–30 μm in diameter), have myelinated processes, represent 90% to 95% of the population, and innervate inner hair cells.
- Type II ganglion cells are small (15–20 μm in diameter), unmyelinated, represent the remainder of the ganglion population, and innervate exclusively outer hair cells.

Cats have approximately 50,000 ganglion cells in each ear.[49] The central axons of the spiral ganglion cells collect within the central core of the cochlea, called the modiolus, and form the cochlear nerve. The cochlear nerve joins with the vestibular nerve to form the vestibulocochlear nerve, which together, along with the facial nerve, occupies the internal acoustic meatus within the petrous portion of the temporal bone. The vestibulocochlear nerve travels toward the brainstem where the cochlear branch enters and terminates within the cochlear nucleus, whereas the vestibular branch passes beneath and around the cochlear nucleus to arch up to the vestibular nuclei.

EFFECTS OF DEAFNESS ON THE AUDITORY SYSTEM

White cats with blue eyes are undoubtedly the best-known representatives of feline deafness. Deafness in white cats has been extensively studied with a number of

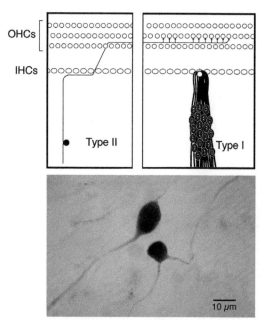

Fig. 6. Receptor innervation by ganglion cells. (*Top*) drawing that illustrates the segregated innervation of hair cells by the 2 types of spiral ganglion cells. Type II neurons represent only 5% to 10% of the population and innervate multiple outer hair cells. In contrast, type I neurons represent the remaining 90% to 95% and innervate exclusively inner hair cells. Each IHC is innervated by 10 to 20 ganglion cells. (*Bottom*) photomicrograph of representative type I and type II ganglion cells as stained by horseradish peroxidase. (*From* Kiang NY, Morest DK, Godfrey DA, et al. Stimulus coding at caudal levels of the cat's auditory nervous system. I. Response characteristics of single units. In: Moller AR, editor. Basic Mechanisms of Hearing. New York: Academic Press; 1973. p. 455–78; with permission.)

scholarly publications on the subject.[5,6,36,50] The most common cause of deafness in these cats is degeneration of the cochlea and saccule, termed cochleo-saccular degeneration (**Fig. 7**). This deafness mimics the Scheibe deformity of humans,[5,51–53] which features early postnatal onset of sensorineural hearing impairment that is transmitted in an autosomal dominant pattern with incomplete penetrance.[5,36,54–56]

- Blue-eyed white cats can have what is called cochleosaccule degeneration, causing profound deafness.
- White cats can also exhibit "spongioform" degeneration of the internal ear, also causing deafness.
- White cats are not necessarily albino cats. White cats can exhibit varying amounts of melanin, whereas albino cats have no melanin. Some white cats are deaf; albino cats are not deaf.

Deaf white cats show an absence of melanocytes,[57] whereas albinos have a normal distribution of melanocytes but lack the enzyme tyrosinase and so are incapable of producing melanin pigment.[58] Although albino cats are not deaf, they exhibit abnormal auditory evoked brainstem responses (ABR) at least when compared with pigmented cats.[59] Although ABR thresholds, peak shapes, and peak latencies can vary considerably from laboratory to laboratory,[60–62] there is a distinct loss of sensitivity in albino

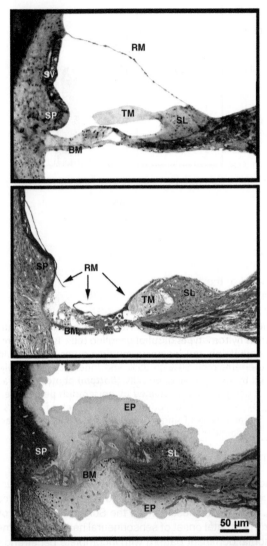

Fig. 7. Photomicrographs of organ of Corti in cats with normal hearing (*top*); cats deafened by the collapse of Reissner membrane, thinning of the stria vascularis, and obliteration of the sensory epithelium (*middle*); and cats deafened by spongioform hypertrophy that destroys the organ of Corti (*bottom*).[65] Scale bar equals 50 μm. BM, basilar membrane; EP, epithelium; RM, Reissner membrane; SL, spiral limbus; SP, spiral prominence; SV, stria vascularis; TM, tectorial membrane. (*From* Ryugo DK, Cahill HB, Rose LS, et al. Separate forms of pathology in the cochlea of congenitally deaf white cats. Hear Res 2003;181:73–84, with permission.)

cats. The underlying causes of these variations are unknown but definite atrophic changes in the auditory pathway occur as a result of pigment-related alterations of internal ear development.[63]

The appearance of the internal ear of deaf cats is strikingly different from that of hearing cats. Cats were given hearing tests when they were 30 days postnatal. At this age, cats with normal hearing stabilize their pinna reflex, orient appropriately to sounds in space, and learn to differentiate between sounds.[64] Moreover, mesenchyme has cleared from the middle ear and the external ear canal is open to the tympanic membrane.[65] Deafness is indicated by a failure to elicit a sound-evoked brain response and is coupled to cochlear pathology. Deafness in white cats was correlated with 2 types of structural abnormalities. The more common form resembled that previously reported[5,6,66,67] in which the Reissner membrane is collapsed on the organ of Corti and the scala media is obliterated (middle panel, see **Fig. 7**). The collapse occurs during the first 10 postnatal days. The stria vascularis is present but is distinctly thinner than normal (compare top and middle panel, see **Fig. 7**). By the time the external ear canal opens (after the third postnatal week), kittens that are completely unresponsive to acoustic stimulation have no scala media on histologic examination. In older deaf cats, the organ of Corti is virtually unrecognizable.

The other form of cochlear pathology in white cats featured a proliferation of cells throughout the cochlear spiral (bottom panel, see **Fig. 7**). There was a hypertrophy of Reissner membrane such that it became highly irregular and folded, eventually filling the scala media.[65] The supporting cells of the organ of Corti and epithelial cells of the basilar membrane hypertrophied as well. The basilar membrane was buckled, the tunnel of Corti never attained its characteristic triangular shape, hair cells did not differentiate, and the stria vascularis was obscured. Overall, the tissue exhibited a "spongiform" appearance.

Spiral ganglion cells have their cell bodies in the peripheral auditory system, but extend their central terminations into the central auditory system. The survival of these ganglion neurons is dependent on the health of the organ of Corti because they undergo degeneration that is associated with hair cell loss and sensorineural deafness.[68–72] In congenitally deaf white cats, there is a gradual loss of spiral ganglion cells with age with about half the ganglion cell population surviving after a year (**Fig. 8**). Several studies have addressed the effects of intracochlear electrical stimulation on spiral ganglion cell survival following neonatal deafness because of the importance these cells play in the outcome of cochlear implants. The actual benefits of electrical stimulation are still subject of debate because of conflicting outcomes.[73–80]

TRANS-SYNAPTIC CHANGES IN THE AUDITORY PATHWAY: COCHLEAR NUCLEUS

Afferent activity is essential for the normal development and maintenance of the central auditory system in mammals. Reductions of cochlear nerve input to the brain have been produced by drugs, nerve section or cochlear ablation, and noise trauma. These measures produce dramatic changes in the structure and function of the central auditory pathway.[81–90] Are the pathologic changes attributable to the side effects of experimental manipulations, missing sensory receptors, absent cochlear nerve activity, or deafness regardless of cause? Does auditory enrichment have an opposing effect on brain structure and function as compared with auditory deprivation? To better understand the "nurture" component of brain development, we need to establish baseline features for the normal central auditory system as well as for the hearing impaired system.

Electrophysiological recordings from cochlear nerve fibers of pigmented cats with normal hearing provided standard tuning curves and thresholds.[67] These cats also exhibited normal startle and orientation responses to hand claps presented behind them. In contrast, deaf white cats exhibit no such behavioral responses, no sound-evoked spike activity, and greatly reduced spontaneous activity. The sampling of fibers was based on intracellular penetration, so we did not bias our results by

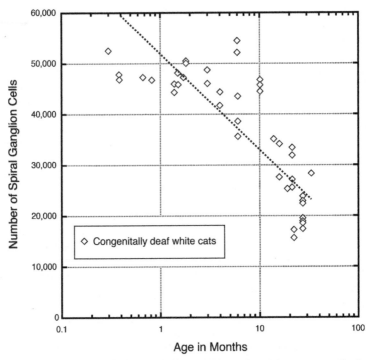

Fig. 8. Plot of spiral ganglion cell loss over time as determined for congenitally deaf white cats. (*Data from* Mair IW. Hereditary deafness in the white cat. Acta Otolaryngol Suppl 1973;314:1–48; and Chen I, Limb CJ, Ryugo DK. The effect of cochlear implant-mediated electrical stimulation on spiral ganglion cells in congenitally deaf white cats. J Assoc Res Otolaryngol 2010;11:587–603.)

searching for the presence of "extracellular" action potentials. The sudden potential drop from 0 to –40 mV indicated that the recording tip of the electrode was "inside" an individual cochlear nerve fiber,[91,92] so fibers with near zero spontaneous activity were not missed.

Activity and Structure

Roughly 60% of cochlear nerve fibers exhibit high levels of spontaneous spike discharges (40–100 spikes per second) in normal hearing cats. It is no wonder that neural activity exerts an influence on cellular morphology. Sensorineural hearing loss results in a loss of activity whose effect on target cell size in the cochlear nucleus can vary among the different cell types.[93–95] The cochlear nucleus is not a homogeneous structure. A number of different neuron populations have been described that are associated with different classes of cochlear nerve endings.[96–99] The idea has been suggested that the relationship between inputs and cell morphology defines the neuron's response to sound.[100,101] What has emerged over the years is the notion that neuron classes can be defined by shared physiologic response properties, morphologic characteristics, and synaptic inputs, and that they form different cell populations that have separate outputs to higher centers. These divergent circuits process different features of sound but converge again at a "central processor" to produce a percept of the auditory signal.

The timing and synchrony of this processing is crucial because continuity is what unifies sounds into a coherent stream. We describe one circuit involved in acoustic "timing" to illustrate this idea. Brain changes caused by peripheral hearing loss must be mediated, at least in part, by cochlear nerve fibers and their interactions in the cochlear nucleus. Because the cochlear nucleus is the gateway to the central auditory system, any corruption of signal processing that occurs there will be felt at higher centers. The pathophysiology manifest at the cochlear nucleus will indicate where else in the auditory system defects might appear.

At the termination of the ascending branch of each cochlear nerve fiber is a prominent axosomatic terminal ending that is distinguished by its large size and complex arborization around the postsynaptic cell body (**Fig. 9**). This distinctive class of synaptic ending is called an endbulb.[99,102,103] Interestingly, in every land vertebrate examined, cochlear nerve fibers terminate in the cochlear nucleus with an endbulb.[104] The evolutionary conservation and large size emphasize its importance to auditory processing. The numerous synaptic release sites that embrace the cell body of a spherical bushy cell suggest a fail-safe transmission from nerve fiber to brain cell, exactly the relationship necessary to preserve timing in the auditory signal. Recall that the ability to localize the source of a sound depends on 2 ears: the ear closer to the source hears the sound sooner and louder than the far ear. The difference in time of arrival and loudness between the 2 ears provides the cues for sound localization. The endbulb and its postsynaptic neuron form the start of the brain circuit that encodes timing.

It had been observed that endbulb morphology was distinctly related to the spontaneous discharge rate (SR) and threshold of the cochlear nerve fiber in normal-hearing cats. Those endbulbs arising from fibers with low activity exhibit smaller but more highly complex arborizations in comparison with those fibers of high activity.[105] This activity-related difference in endbulb morphology is subtle and required fractal analysis to provide conclusive evidence of this variation. In the cats with hearing loss, analysis revealed endbulb size and branching complexity to be correlated with hearing sensitivity and fiber activity (**Fig. 10**).

Endbulb Synapses

Differences in endbulb branching complexity were observed as a reflection of hearing status. Endbulb synapses were then examined with the aid of an electron microscope because synapses represent the crucial functional unit. Cochlear nerve synapses from normal-hearing cats have been well described,[106,107] so they will be only briefly

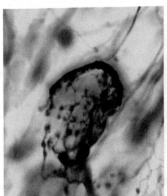 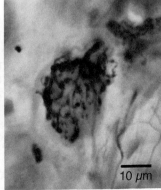

10 μm

Fig. 9. Photomicrographs of typical endbulbs stained by horseradish peroxidase in the cochlear nucleus of the cat. Note their large size and elaborate branching pattern. A cell body is nestled within the grasp of the endbulb arborization. (*Courtesy of* Dr David K. Ryugo, Garvan Institute of Medical Research, Sydney, Australia.)

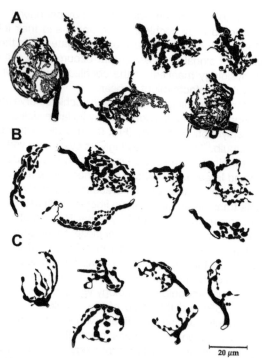

Fig. 10. Camera lucida drawings of endbulbs from normal-hearing cat (*A*), white cat with 50 dB hearing loss (*B*), and congenitally deaf white cat (*C*). Note that the complexity of the shape of endbulbs diminishes with hearing loss. (*From* Ryugo DK, Rosenbaum BT, Kim PJ, et al. Single unit recordings in the auditory nerve of congenitally deaf white cats: morphologic correlates in the cochlea and cochlear nucleus. J Comp Neurol 1998;397:532–48; with permission.)

mentioned for comparison purposes with those of the white cats. Transmitter release sites form around discrete postsynaptic densities, where the postsynaptic membrane bulges into the presynaptic endbulb to form a dome (**Fig. 11**). Clear, round synaptic vesicles are scattered throughout the endbulb cytoplasm but are concentrated around the release sites. A normal endbulb may have up to 2000 individual presynaptic release sites,[108] which oppose round-to-oval membrane thickenings called the postsynaptic density (PSD). These membrane specializations contain transmitter receptors and are distributed relatively uniformly beneath the overlying endbulb.

In contrast, synapses from totally deaf white cats appear distinctly different. Presynaptic vesicle density is distinctly increased and postsynaptic densities are thicker and considerably expanded (**Fig. 12**). Reconstructing the postsynaptic membrane, which lays beneath the presynaptic endbulb, demonstrated PSD hypertrophy by its expansion over the surface of the neuron. Synapses of partially deaf cats (eg, those with elevated thresholds), however, seemed to represent a transition between normal and deaf synapses.[67]

TRANS-SYNAPTIC CHANGES IN THE AUDITORY PATHWAY: SUPERIOR OLIVARY COMPLEX

The medial superior olive (MSO) is the first site in the central auditory pathway where convergence of neural information from the 2 ears occurs (**Fig. 13**). The convergence arises from the cochlear nucleus neurons that are the recipients of endbulb synapses.

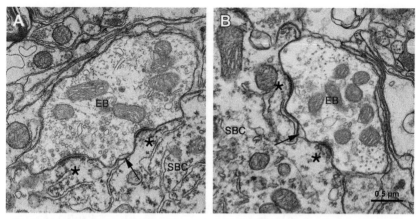

Fig. 11. Electron micrographs through synapses of endbulbs (EB) from cats with normal hearing.[134] The endbulb (*yellow*) forms synapses opposite dome-shaped postsynaptic densities (*asterisk*) and round synaptic vesicles accumulate along the presynaptic membrane. Cisternae (*arrow*) form between the membrane of the endbulb and that of the postsynaptic spherical bushy cell (SBC); these intermembraneous channels may serve as "gutters" to facilitate transmitter diffusion away from the synapse. Scale bar equals 0.5 μm. (*From* O'Neil JN, Limb CJ, Baker CA, et al. Bilateral effects of unilateral cochlear implantation in congenitally deaf cats. J Comp Neurol 2010;518:2382–404, with permission.)

The principal neurons of the MSO are aligned in a vertical sheet with its diametrically opposed bipolar dendrites facing medially and laterally.[109] Excitatory inputs are segregated such that ipsilateral input innervates lateral dendrites in the ipsilateral MSO and medial dendrites of the contralateral MSO.[110,111] These neurons have a proposed function as a "coincidence detector" for processing interaural timing differences (ITD).[112] In addition, inhibitory inputs to the MSO arise from the medial (MNTB) and lateral

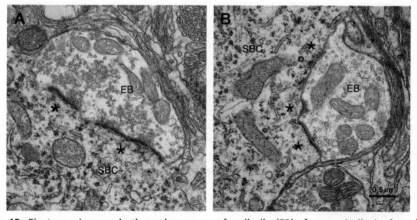

Fig. 12. Electron micrographs through synapses of endbulbs (EB) of congenitally deaf cats.[135] The postsynaptic densities of these synapses have hypertrophied (*asterisk*) and become more flattened. Synaptic vesicles have proliferated in the endbulb (*yellow*) cytoplasm and intermembraneous channels have disappeared. The scale bar equals 0.5 μm. (*From* O'Neil JN, Limb CJ, Baker CA, et al. Bilateral effects of unilateral cochlear implantation in congenitally deaf cats. J Comp Neurol 2010;518:2382–404, with permission.)

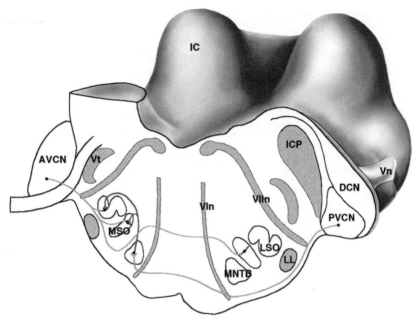

Fig. 13. Caudal-lateral view of the cat brain stem where the cut surface passes through the superior olivary complex. The cut is angled so that it also passes through different parts of the cochlear nucleus on the left and right. The excitatory path from the spherical bushy cells of the left anteroventral cochlear nucleus (AVCN) initiates processing of interaural timing differences in the medial superior olive (MSO) and interaural level differences in the lateral superior olive (LSO). The excitatory path from globular bushy cells of the right posteroventral cochlear nucleus (PVCN) initiates the processing of interaural level differences, and its target is the medial nucleus of the trapezoid body (MNTB). The output of the MNTB is inhibitory (*red*) and it terminates in the MSO and LSO. AVCN, anteroventral cochlear nucleus; DCN, dorsal cochlear nucleus; IC, inferior colliculus; ICP, inferior cerebellar peduncle; LL, lateral lemniscus; LSO, lateral superior olive; MNTB, medial nucleus of the trapezoid body; MSO, medial superior olive; VIn, abducens (sixth) nerve root; VIIn, facial (seventh) nerve root; Vn, trigeminal (fifth) cranial nerve; Vt, spinal trigeminal tract. (*Courtesy of* Catherine Connelly, Garvan Institute of Medical Research, Sydney, Australia.)

nucleus of the trapezoid body (LNTB), are confined to the cell bodies of MSO neurons, and function to adjust the output signal of MSO neurons to higher centers.[113,114]

Congenital deafness causes a bilateral disruption in the spatially segregated inputs to the MSO principal neurons such that inhibitory input at the cell body is significantly reduced compared with what is observed in hearing animals.[90,111] This change in axosomatic inhibition was manifest by a loss of staining for gephyrin, an anchoring protein for the glycine receptor,[111] and the migration of terminals containing flattened and pleomorphic synaptic vesicles (indicative of inhibitory synapses) away from the cell body.[90] Excitatory inputs to the dendrites were severely shrunken[90] and the dendrites themselves atrophied.[115]

TRANS-SYNAPTIC CHANGES IN THE AUDITORY PATHWAY: INFERIOR COLLICULUS

The inferior colliculus (IC) is a complex, tonotopically organized nucleus of the midbrain receiving auditory inputs from many ascending brainstem sources including both cochlear nuclei, superior olivary complex, and nuclei of the lateral lemniscus, as well as descending inputs from the auditory cortex and superior colliculus.[116–118] It is a large bilateral nucleus. A rudimentary tonotopic organization within the IC has been shown to exist in long-term deafened animals.[119,120] This organization is evident even in congenitally deaf animals, implying that a blueprint for connections is in place and can develop even without the benefit of hearing.[121]

Acute deafness did not increase temporal dispersion in spike timing to trains of electric pulse stimulation in the cochlear nerve nor impair ITD sensitivity.[122,123] Congenital deafness, however, did reduce ITD sensitivity in the responses of IC units. Single-cell recordings in the IC showed that half as many neurons in the congenitally deaf cat showed ITD sensitivity to electrical stimulation when compared with the acutely deafened animals. In neurons that showed ITD tuning, they were found to be broad and variable.[124] The synaptic changes that disrupt the electrophysiological response properties are a reflection of neuronal response profiles that arise from lower structures in the pathway.[125–128] Collectively, the data imply that ITD discrimination is a highly demanding process and that even with near perfect synapse restoration, the task is sufficiently difficult that perhaps only complete restoration of synapses will enable the full return of function.

TRANS-SYNAPTIC CHANGES IN THE AUDITORY PATHWAY: AUDITORY CORTEX

The end point of stimulus coding along the auditory pathway presumably occurs in the auditory areas of the cerebral cortex. Acoustic features, such as distance, location,

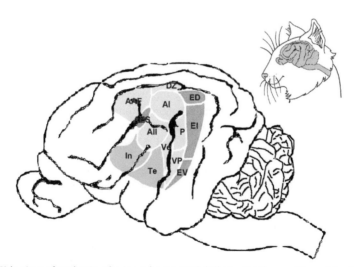

Fig. 14. Side view of cat brain. The inset (*upper right*) illustrates the position of the brain relative to the head. The gyral patterns of the cortex are fairly reproducible across individual cats but they are not identical; thus, they are not reliable markers for cortical function. The many auditory areas reflect the complex processing involved in creating sound awareness. AAF, anterior auditory field; AES, anterior ectosylvian sulcus area; AI, primary auditory cortex; AII, secondary auditory cortex; DZ, dorsal auditory zone; ED, posterior ectosylvian gyrus; EI, posterior ectosylvian gyrus, intermediate part; EV, posterior ectosylvian gyrus, ventral part; in, insular cortex; P, auditory cortex, posterior area; Te, temporal cortex; Ve, auditory cortex, ventral area; VP, auditory cortex, ventral posterior area. (*Courtesy of* David K. Ryugo, Garvan Institute of Medical Research, Sydney, Australia; *data from* Winer JA, Lee CC. The distributed auditory cortex. Hear Res 2007;229:3–13.)

pitch, motion, and significance, are carried by the auditory stream and become unified into a single percept. This unity is coordinated by a system of multiple auditory areas that are fed by the parallel sets of ascending pathways. Hierarchically processed acoustic events are distributed across the different cortical areas and assembled for cognitive interpretation (**Fig. 14**). The number and complexity of cortical areas is testament to the computational demands on hearing.[129] Not surprisingly, congenital deafness leads to functional and morphologic abnormalities along the auditory pathway, including auditory cortex.[130,131] The repair of these defects, fortunately, can be achieved through the timely restoration of normal activity in the auditory system.[132–134]

SUMMARY

In summary, hearing is a vital sense in the everyday life of cats. It enables them to be constantly aware of their environment, especially when vision is insufficient. Hearing loss represents a huge disadvantage to them, and there are many possible sources of this disability. Deafness can be a result of genetic mutation, disease, industrial noise, ototoxic chemicals, or trauma. Any of these sources could cause abnormalities in sensory transduction in the ear that lead to brain pathology in structure, chemistry, synaptic transmission, or perceptual dysfunction owing to fouled circuits. Regardless of the cause, sensorineural deafness produces change in many parts of the nervous system that in general, cannot be treated, but contribute to the pathology.

GLOSSARY

ABR: ABR is the acronym for a sound-evoked auditory brainstem response. It is a noninvasive means of assessing auditory responses of the brain as recorded from the scalp. Because of the relatively large distance from recording site to brain, the response must be averaged over 500 to 1000 stimulus presentations.

Action potential, membrane potential: Action potential refers to a rapid change in electrical potential that is measured between the inside and outside of a nerve or muscle cell when stimulated. It is the common unit of communication between nerve cells.

Afferent: Afferent is a term used to describe individual neurons, systems of neurons, or parts of neurons that convey information toward another neuron or into the central nervous system.

Arborization: Arborization is a term used to describe a "treelike" appearance of certain neuron outgrowths, either an axon or its termination or the shape of dendritic branching.

Autosomal dominant locus: Autosome refers to any chromosome that is not a sex-determining chromosome (eg, not X and not Y). Two copies of every gene are located on a chromosome and tend to work together; when one gene over-powers the other, it is said to be dominant. The locus refers to the gene's specific location on an identified chromosome.

Axosomatic: Axosomatic refers to the relationship between an incoming synaptic terminal and the postsynaptic target, where "axo" refers to the incoming presyn-aptic structure and "somatic" indicates the postsynaptic cell body or soma. In this case, the axon terminal forms a synapse on the cell body of the target neuron. Axodendritic describes the case in which an incoming axon terminal synapses on the dendrite. And so on.

Candidate gene approach: The candidate gene approach focuses on associations between genetic variation within specified genes of interest and phenotypic expression of disease state or trait.

Central auditory system: The central auditory system is that part of the hearing system that resides within the brain. It is composed of many neuronal structures that are linked together by axonal pathways to form an integrated system. Its normal function is to convert the physical attributes of sound into conscious perceptions of auditory meaning.

Cochleosaccule dysplasia: Cochleosaccule dysplasia is pathology of the saccule (vestibular sensory organ) and cochlea (hearing organ). The dysplasia is characterized by a collapse of the saccular membrane and Reissner membrane, respectively, onto the sensory epithelium.

Efferent: Efferent is the term used to describe individual neurons, systems of neurons, or parts of neurons that convey information away from its origin, as away from the cell body or away from the central nervous system.

Endolymph, endolymphatic space, endocochlear potential: Endolymph is the specialized fluid of the inner ear that bathes the organ of Corti. It is contained within the endolymphatic space, which is equivalent to the cochlear duct. Its special high potassium content endows it with a positive potential (approximately +80 mV) relative to ground; the potential is called the endocochlear potential.

Gap junctions: Gap junctions are membrane specializations between 2 cells that allow electrical coupling and the passage of ions and small molecules. These specializations underlie electrical synapses.

Gloving: The gloving gene is implicated in the white feet of pigmented cats.

Interaural time disparity: Interaural time disparity refers to the circumstance in which a sound located away from the listener's midline arrives at the closer ear before it arrives at the farther ear. The difference in time of arrival is computed by the brain to inform the organism where along the horizontal plane, with respect to the head, the sound originated.

KIT: Kit is a gene that is involved in the production of melanocytes, blood cells, mast cells, and stem cells. Mutations of this gene are known to cause white coat color.

Knockouts: Knockouts or gene knockouts refer to a genetically engineered mouse in which a gene has been inactivated or deleted ("knocked out").

Linkage: Linkage is the tendency of genes that are located near each other on a chromosome to be inherited together. The probability of such an occurrence is calculated by testing if the 2 loci are linked compared with observing the same traits purely by chance.

Melanocytes: Melanocytes are neural-crest–derived, melanin-producing cells found mainly in the epidermis but also in eyes, ears, and meninges.

Mesenchyme: Mesenchyme refers to cells of mesodermal origin that are capable of developing into connective tissue, blood, or endothelial tissue.

Myelinated: Myelin is an insulating sheath around individual axons formed by the tight wrapping of cell membrane of oligodendrocytes in the central nervous system and Schwann cells in the peripheral nervous system.

Peripheral auditory system: The peripheral auditory system is that part of the hearing apparatus that resides in the cochlea (or inner ear).

Pitch: Pitch is related to the frequency of sound vibrations and is an attribute of auditory sensation whereby sounds may be ordered from low to high.

Pleiotropic effects: Pleiotropic refers to having multiple effects from a single gene.

Pleomorphic synaptic vesicles: Pleomorphic synaptic vesicles is the term used to describe the circumstance in which synaptic vesicles in aldehyde-preserved tissue, when examined with an electron microscope, exhibit a variety of shapes from round to oval to flattened. This variety of vesicle shapes is inferred to indicate inhibitory action at the associated synapse.

Potential difference: Potential difference refers to the voltage difference between 2 points. In the case of endolymph and perilymph, it reflects the differential distribution of Na+, K+, and Cl– within 2 closed compartments.

Receptor cell: Receptor cells are specialized to convert energy in the form of light, chemical, or mechanical into neural signals.

Spongiform: Spongiform is an adjective used to describe the spongelike appearance of a pathologic overgrowth of cells in the cochlea.

Spontaneous discharge rate: Spontaneous discharge rate refers to the situation in which a neuron gives rise to action potentials in the absence of experimenter-delivered stimulation.

Stereocilia: Stereocilia are specialized microvilli that form on the top surface of auditory and vestibular sensory receptor cells. Deformation of the stereocilia in one direction opens ion channels, whereas deformation in the opposite direction closes them.

Synapse: The synapse is a structure at the point of communication between 2 neurons where chemical or electrical signals can be passed.

Syndromic deafness, nonsyndromic deafness: Syndromic deafness refers to hearing loss that is associated with other distinctive medical conditions; nonsyndromic deafness occurs by itself.

Tonotopic: Tonotopic is a term used to describe the systematic organization of frequency across an auditory structure, where there is a progression of frequency representation from low to high.

W: The primary gene responsible for white color. It is dominant over other colors, so white cats can be either Ww or WW. Cats that are ww express pigmentation patterns determined by other genes.

Waardenburg syndrome: Waardenburg syndrome is a group of inherited conditions passed down through families that involve deafness and pale skin, hair, and eye color.

ACKNOWLEDGMENTS

The authors are grateful for the published data of their colleagues that made this review possible, and to Karen Henoch-Ryugo and Bradley L. Njaa for editorial comments on earlier drafts. The content of this publication does not necessarily reflect the views or policies of the Department of Health and Human Services or the National Health and Medical Research Council, nor does mention of trade names, commercial products, or organizations imply endorsement by the US or Australian governments.

REFERENCES

1. Liberman MC. Auditory-nerve response from cats raised in a low-noise chamber. J Acoust Soc Am 1978;63:442–55.
2. Pickles JO. An introduction to the physiology of hearing. Bingley (United Kingdom): Emerald; 2008.
3. Darwin C. The Origin of Species: 150th Anniversary Edition. New York: New American Library; 1859 republished in 2003.
4. Tait L. Note on deafness in white cats. Nature 1883;29:164.

5. Bosher S, Hallpike C. Observations on the histological features, development and pathogenesis of the inner ear degeneration of the deaf white cat. Proc R Soc Lond B Biol Sci 1965;162:147–70.
6. Mair IW. Hereditary deafness in the white cat. Acta Otolaryngol Suppl 1973;314: 1–48.
7. Chabot B, Stephenson DA, Chapman VM, et al. The proto-oncogene c-kit encoding a transmembrane tyrosine kinase receptor maps to the mouse W locus. Nature 1988;335:88–9.
8. Clark LA, Wahl JM, Rees CA, et al. Retrotransposon insertion in SILV is responsible for merle patterning of the domestic dog. Proc Natl Acad Sci U S A 2006; 103:1376–81.
9. Flottorp G, Foss I. Development of hearing in hereditarily deaf white mink (Hedlund) and normal mink (standard) and the subsequent deterioration of the auditory response in Hedlund mink. Acta Otolaryngol 1979;87:16–27.
10. Gauly M, Vaughan J, Hogreve SK, et al. Brainstem auditory-evoked potential assessment of auditory function and congenital deafness in llamas (*Lama glama*) and alpacas (*L. pacos*). J Vet Intern Med 2005;19:756–60.
11. Haase B, Brooks SA, Schlumbaum A, et al. Allelic heterogeneity at the equine KIT locus in dominant white (W) horses. PLoS Genet 2007;3:e195.
12. Haase B, Brooks SA, Tozaki T, et al. Seven novel KIT mutations in horses with white coat colour phenotypes. Anim Genet 2009;40:623–9.
13. Hilding DA, Sugiura A, Nakai Y. Deaf white mink: electron microscopic study of the inner ear. Ann Otol Rhinol Laryngol 1967;76:647–63.
14. Hodgkinson CA, Nakayama A, Li H, et al. Mutation at the anophthalmic white locus in Syrian hamsters: haploinsufficiency in the Mitf gene mimics human Waardenburg syndrome type 2. Hum Mol Genet 1998;7:703–8.
15. Hudson W, Ruben R. Hereditary deafness in the Dalmation dog. Arch Otolaryngol 1962;75:213–9.
16. Karlsson EK, Baranowska I, Wade CM, et al. Efficient mapping of mendelian traits in dogs through genome-wide association. Nat Genet 2007;39: 1321–8.
17. Magdesian KG, Williams DC, Aleman M, et al. Evaluation of deafness in American Paint horses by phenotype, brainstem auditory-evoked responses, and endothelin receptor B genotype. J Am Vet Med Assoc 2009;235:1204–11.
18. Ruan HB, Zhang N, Gao X. Identification of a novel point mutation of mouse proto-oncogene c-kit through N-ethyl-N-nitrosourea mutagenesis. Genetics 2005;169:819–31.
19. Tsujimura T, Hirota S, Nomura S, et al. Characterization of Ws mutant allele of rats: a 12-base deletion in tyrosine kinase domain of c-kit gene. Blood 1991; 78:1942–6.
20. Silvers WK. The coat colors of mice: a model for mammalian gene action and interaction. New York: Springer-Verlag; 1979.
21. Epstein DJ, Vekemans M, Gros P. Splotch (Sp2H), a mutation affecting development of the mouse neural tube, shows a deletion within the paired homeodomain of Pax-3. Cell 1991;67:767–74.
22. Tachibana M, Hara Y, Vyas D, et al. Cochlear disorder associated with melanocyte anomaly in mice with a transgenic insertional mutation. Mol Cell Neurosci 1992;3:433–45.
23. Hodgkinson CA, Moore KJ, Nakayama A, et al. Mutations at the mouse microphthalmia locus are associated with defects in a gene encoding a novel basic-helix-loop-helix-zipper protein. Cell 1993;74:395–404.

24. Baynash AG, Hosoda K, Giaid A, et al. Interaction of endothelin-3 with endothelin-B receptor is essential for development of epidermal melanocytes and enteric neurons. Cell 1994;79:1277–85.

25. Tachibana M, Perez-Jurado LA, Nakayama A, et al. Cloning of MITF, the human homolog of the mouse microphthalmia gene and assignment to chromosome 3p14.1-p12.3. Hum Mol Genet 1994;3:553–7.

26. Attie T, Till M, Pelet A, et al. Mutation of the endothelin-receptor B gene in Waardenburg-Hirschsprung disease. Hum Mol Genet 1995;4:2407–9.

27. Southard-Smith EM, Kos L, Pavan WJ. Sox10 mutation disrupts neural crest development in Dom Hirschsprung mouse model. Nat Genet 1998;18:60–4.

28. Syrris P, Carter ND, Patton MA. Novel nonsense mutation of the endothelin-B receptor gene in a family with Waardenburg-Hirschsprung disease. Am J Med Genet 1999;87:69–71.

29. Herbarth B, Pingault V, Bondurand N, et al. Mutation of the Sry-related Sox10 gene in Dominant megacolon, a mouse model for human Hirschsprung disease. Proc Natl Acad Sci U S A 1998;95:5161–5.

30. Sanchez-Martin M, Rodriguez-Garcia A, Perez-Losada J, et al. SLUG (SNAI2) deletions in patients with Waardenburg disease. Hum Mol Genet 2002;11: 3231–6.

31. Tasaki I, Spyropoulos CS. Stria vascularis as source of endocochlear potential. J Neurophysiol 1959;22:149–55.

32. Marcus DC, Wu T, Wangemann P, et al. KCNJ10 (Kir4.1) potassium channel knockout abolishes endocochlear potential. Am J Physiol Cell Physiol 2002; 282:C403–7.

33. Geigy CA, Heid S, Steffen F, et al. Does a pleiotropic gene explain deafness and blue irises in white cats? Vet J 2007;173:548–53.

34. Mullikin JC, Hansen NF, Shen L, et al. Light whole genome sequence for SNP discovery across domestic cat breeds. BMC Genomics 2010;11:406.

35. Menotti-Raymond M, David VA, Pflueger S, et al. Widespread retinal degenerative disease mutation (rdAc) discovered among a large number of popular cat breeds. Vet J 2010;186:32–8.

36. Bergsma D, Brown K. White fur, blue eyes, and deafness in the domestic cat. J Hered 1971;62:171–85.

37. Aoki H, Yamada Y, Hara A, et al. Two distinct types of mouse melanocyte: differential signaling requirement for the maintenance of non-cutaneous and dermal versus epidermal melanocytes. Development 2009;136:2511–21.

38. Cooper MP, Fretwell N, Bailey SJ, et al. White spotting in the domestic cat (*Felis catus*) maps near KIT on feline chromosome B1. Anim Genet 2006;37:163–5.

39. Lyons LA. Feline genetics: clinical applications and genetic testing. Top Companion Anim Med 2010;25:203–12.

40. Dallos P. Overview: cochlear neurobiology. In: Dallos P, Popper AN, Fay RR, editors. The cochlea. New York: Springer; 1996. p. 1–43.

41. Wangemann P. K$^+$ cycling and the endocochlear potential. Hear Res 2002; 165:1–9.

42. Wangemann P, Schacht J. Homeostasic mechanisms in the cochlea. In: Dallos P, Popper AN, Fay RR, editors. The cochlea. New York: Springer; 1996. p. 130–85.

43. Cohen-Salmon M, Regnault B, Cayet N, et al. Connexin30 deficiency causes instrastrial fluid-blood barrier disruption within the cochlear stria vascularis. Proc Natl Acad Sci U S A 2007;104:6229–34.

44. Rhys Evans PH, Comis SD, Osborne MP, et al. Cross-links between stereocilia in the human organ of Corti. J Laryngol Otol 1985;99:11–9.

45. Pickles JO, Comis SD, Osborne MP. Cross-links between stereocilia in the guinea pig organ of Corti, and their possible relation to sensory transduction. Hear Res 1984;15:103–12.

46. Dallos P. The active cochlea. J Neurosci 1992;12:4575–85.

47. Spoendlin H. The innervation of the cochlea receptor. In: Moller AR, editor. Mechanisms in hearing. New York: Academic Press; 1973. p. 185–229.

48. Kiang NY, Rho JM, Northrop CC, et al. Hair-cell innervation by spiral ganglion cells in adult cats. Science 1982;217:175–7.

49. Chen I, Limb CJ, Ryugo DK. The effect of cochlear implant-mediated electrical stimulation on spiral ganglion cells in congenitally deaf white cats. J Assoc Res Otolaryngol 2010;11:587–603.

50. Strain GM. Deafness in dogs and cats. Wallingford (CT): CABI; 2011.

51. Deol MS. The relationship between abnormalities of pigmentation and of the inner ear. Proc R Soc Lond B Biol Sci 1970;175:201–17.

52. Suga F, Hattler KW. Physiological and histopathological correlates of hereditary deafness in animals. Laryngoscope 1970;80:81–104.

53. Brighton P, Ramesar R, Winship I. Hearing impairment and pigmentary disturbance. Ann N Y Acad Sci 1991;630:152–66.

54. Rawitz B. Gehörorgan und gehirn eines weissen Hundes mit blauen Augen. Morphol Arbeit 1896;6:545–54.

55. Wolff D. Three generations of deaf white cats. J Hered 1942;33:39–43.

56. Bosher SK, Hallpike CS. Observations on the histogenesis of the inner ear degeneration of the deaf white cat and its possible relationship to the aetiology of certain unexplained varieties of human congenital deafness. J Laryngol Otol 1966;80:222–35.

57. Billingham RE, Silvers WK. The melanocytes of mammals. Q Rev Biol 1960;35: 1–40.

58. Imes DL, Geary LA, Grahn RA, et al. Albinism in the domestic cat (Felis catus) is associated with a tyrosinase (TYR) mutation. Anim Genet 2006;37:175–8.

59. Creel D, Conlee JW, Parks TN. Auditory brainstem anomalies in albino cats. I. Evoked potential studies. Brain Res 1983;260:1–9.

60. Buchwald JS, Huang CM. Far-Field acoustic response: origins in the cat. Science 1975;189:382–4.

61. Berry H, Blair RL, Bilbao J, et al. Click evoked eighth nerve and brain stem responses (electrocochleogram)—experimental observations in the cat. J Otolaryngol 1976;5:64–73.

62. Achor LJ, Starr A. Auditory brain stem responses in the cat. I. Intracranial and extracranial recordings. Electroencephalogr Clin Neurophysiol 1980;48:154–73.

63. Conlee JW, Parks TN, Romero C, et al. Auditory brainstem anomalies in albino cats: II. Neuronal atrophy in the superior olive. J Comp Neurol 1984;225:141–8.

64. Villablanca JR, Olmstead CE. Neurological development in kittens. Dev Psychobiol 1979;12:101–27.

65. Ryugo DK, Cahill HB, Rose LS, et al. Separate forms of pathology in the cochlea of congenitally deaf white cats. Hear Res 2003;181:73–84.

66. Rebillard M, Pujol R, Rebillard G. Variability of the hereditary deafness in the white cat. II. Histology. Hear Res 1981;5:189–200.

67. Ryugo DK, Rosenbaum BT, Kim PJ, et al. Single unit recordings in the auditory nerve of congenitally deaf white cats: morphological correlates in the cochlea and cochlear nucleus. J Comp Neurol 1998;397:532–48.

68. Webster M, Webster DB. Spiral ganglion neuron loss following organ of Corti loss: a quantitative study. Brain Res 1981;212:17–30.

69. Spoendlin H. Factors inducing retrograde degeneration of the cochlear nerve. Ann Otol Rhinol Laryngol 1984;112(Suppl):76–82.

70. Leake PA, Hradek GT. Cochlear pathology of long term neomycin induced deafness in cats. Hear Res 1988;33:11–34.

71. Hardie NA, Shepherd RK. Sensorineural hearing loss during development: morphological and physiological response of the cochlea and auditory brainstem. Hear Res 1999;128:147–65.

72. Shepherd RK, Meltzer NE, Fallon JB, et al. Consequences of deafness and electrical stimulation on the peripheral and central auditory system. In: Waltzman SB, Roland JT, editors. Cochlear implants. New York: Thieme Medical Publishers Inc; 2006. p. 25–39.

73. Lousteau RJ. Increased spiral ganglion cell survival in electrically stimulated, deafened guinea pig cochleae. Laryngoscope 1987;97:836–42.

74. Leake PA, Hradek GT, Rebscher SJ, et al. Chronic intracochlear electrical stimulation induces selective survival of spiral ganglion neurons in neonatally deaffened cats. Hear Res 1991;54:251–71.

75. Leake PA, Hradek GT, Snyder RL. Chronic electrical stimulation by a cochlear implant promotes survival of spiral ganglion neurons after neonatal deafness. J Comp Neurol 1999;412:543–62.

76. Leake PA, Stakhovskaya O, Hradek GT, et al. Factors influencing neurotrophic effects of electrical stimulation in the deafened developing auditory system. Hear Res 2008;242:86–99.

77. Araki S, Kawano A, Seldon L, et al. Effects of chronic electrical stimulation on spiral ganglion neuron survival and size in deafened kittens. Laryngoscope 1998;108:687–95.

78. Li L, Parkins CW, Webster DB. Does electrical stimulation of deaf cochleae prevent spiral ganglion degeneration? Hear Res 1999;133:27–39.

79. Shepherd RK, Matsushima J, Martin RL, et al. Cochlear pathology following chronic electrical stimulation of the auditory nerve: II. Deafened kittens. Hear Res 1994;81:150–66.

80. Coco A, Epp SB, Fallon JB, et al. Does cochlear implantation and electrical stimulation affect residual hair cells and spiral ganglion neurons? Hear Res 2007; 225:60–70.

81. Powell TP, Erulkar SD. Transneuronal cell degeneration in the auditory relay nuclei of the cat. J Anat 1962;96:219–68.

82. West CD, Harrison JM. Transneuronal cell atrophy in the deaf white cat. J Comp Neurol 1973;151:377–98.

83. Parks TN. Afferent influences on the development of the brain stem auditory nuclei of the chicken: otocyst ablation. J Comp Neurol 1979;183: 665–77.

84. Nordeen KW, Killackey HP, Kitzes LM. Ascending projections to the inferior colliculus following unilateral cochlear ablation in the neonatal gerbil, *Meriones unguiculatus*. J Comp Neurol 1983;214:144–53.

85. Moore DR, Kowalchuk NE. Auditory brainstem of the ferret: effects of unilateral cochlear lesions on cochlear nucleus volume and projections to the inferior colliculus. J Comp Neurol 1988;272:503–15.

86. Hardie NA, Martsi-McClintock A, Aitkin LM, et al. Neonatal sensorineural hearing loss affects synaptic density in the auditory midbrain. Neuroreport 1998;9: 2019–22.

87. Kral A, Hartmann R, Tillein J, et al. Hearing after congenital deafness: central auditory plasticity and sensory deprivation. Cereb Cortex 2002;12:797–807.

88. Harris JA, Hardie NA, Bermingham-McDonogh O, et al. Gene expression differences over a critical period of afferent-dependent neuron survival in the mouse auditory brainstem. J Comp Neurol 2005;493:460–74.

89. Müller M, Smolders JW. Shift in the cochlear place—frequency map after noise damage in the mouse. Neuroreport 2005;16:1183–7.

90. Tirko NN, Ryugo DK. Synaptic plasticity in the medial superior olive of hearing, deaf, and cochlear-implanted cats. J Comp Neurol 2012;520:2202–17.

91. Liberman MC. Single neuron labelling in the cat auditory nerve. Science 1982b; 216:1239–41.

92. Fekete DM, Rouiller EM, Liberman MC, et al. The central projections of intracellularly labeled auditory nerve fibers in cats. J Comp Neurol 1984;229:432–50.

93. Saada AA, Niparko JK, Ryugo DK. Morphological changes in the cochlear nucleus of congenitally deaf white cats. Brain Res 1996;736:315–28.

94. Redd EE, Pongstaporn T, Ryugo DK. The effects of congenital deafness on auditory nerve synapses and globular bushy cells in cats. Hear Res 2000; 147:160–74.

95. Redd EE, Cahill HB, Pongstaporn T, et al. The effects of congenital deafness on auditory nerve synapses: Type I and Type II multipolar cells in the anteroventral cochlear nucleus of cats. J Assoc Res Otolaryngol 2002;3:403–17.

96. Osen KK. Cytoarchitecture of the cochlear nuclei in the cat. J Comp Neurol 1969;136:453–82.

97. Brawer JR, Morest DK, Kane EC. The neuronal architecture of the cochlear nucleus of the cat. J Comp Neurol 1974;155:251–300.

98. Perkins RE, Morest DK. A study of cochlear innervation patterns in cats and rats with the Golgi method and Nomarkski Optics. J Comp Neurol 1975;163:129–58.

99. Lorente de Nó R. The primary acoustic nuclei. New York: Raven Press; 1981.

100. Kiang NY, Morest DK, Godfrey DA, et al. Stimulus coding at caudal levels of the cat's auditory nervous system. I. Response characteristics of single units. In: Moller AR, editor. Basic mechanisms of hearing. New York: Academic Press; 1973. p. 455–78.

101. Morest DK, Kiang NY, Kane EC, et al. Stimulus coding at caudal levels of the cat's auditory nervous system. II. Pattern of synaptic organization. In: Moller AR, editor. Basic mechanisms of hearing. New York: Academic Press; 1973. p. 479–504.

102. Held H. Die centrale Gehörleitung. Arch Anat Physiol Anat Abt 1893;201–48 [in German].

103. Brawer JR, Morest DK. Relations between auditory nerve endings and cell types in the cat's anteroventral cochlear nucleus seen with the Golgi method and Nomarski optics. J Comp Neurol 1975;160:491–506.

104. Ryugo DK, Parks TN. Primary innervation of the avian and mammalian cochlear nucleus. Brain Res Bull 2003;60:435–56.

105. Sento S, Ryugo DK. Endbulbs of held and spherical bushy cells in cats: morphological correlates with physiological properties. J Comp Neurol 1989; 280:553–62.

106. Lenn NJ, Reese TS. The fine structure of nerve endings in the nucleus of the trapezoid body and the ventral cochlear nucleus. Am J Anat 1966;118: 375–90.

107. Cant NB, Morest DK. The bushy cells in the anteroventral cochlear nucleus of the cat. A study with the electron microscope. Neurosci 1979;4:1925–45.

108. Ryugo DK, Wu MM, Pongstaporn T. Activity-related features of synapse morphology: a study of endbulbs of held. J Comp Neurol 1996;365:141–58.

109. Ramón Y, Cajal R. Histologie du Système Nerveux de l'Homme et des Vertébrés. Madrid: Instituto Ramón y Cajal; 1909.

110. Russell FA, Moore DR. Afferent reorganization within the superior olivary complex of the gerbil: development and induction by neonatal, unilateral cochlear removal. J Comp Neurol 1995;352:607–25.

111. Kapfer C, Seidl AH, Schweizer H, et al. Experience-dependent refinement of inhibitory inputs to auditory coincidence-detector neurons. Nat Neurosci 2002; 5:247–53.

112. Carr CE. Timing is everything: organization of timing circuits in auditory and electrical sensory systems. J Comp Neurol 2004;472:131–3.

113. Grothe B, Sanes DH. Bilateral inhibition by glycinergic afferents in the medial superior olive. J Neurophysiol 1993;69:1192–6.

114. Pecka M, Brand A, Behrend O, et al. Interaural time difference processing in the mammalian medial superior olive: the role of glycinergic inhibition. J Neurosci 2008;28:6914–25.

115. Russell FA, Moore DR. Ultrastructural transynaptic effects of unilateral cochlear ablation in the gerbil medial superior olive. Hear Res 2002;173:43–61.

116. Adams JC. Ascending projections to the inferior colliculus. J Comp Neurol 1979; 183:519–38.

117. Brunso-Bechtold JK, Thompson GC, Masterton RB. HRP study of the organization of auditory afferents ascending to central nucleus of inferior colliculus in cat. J Comp Neurol 1981;197:705–22.

118. Malmierca MS, Ryugo DK. Descending connections to the midbrain and brainstem. In: Winer JA, Schreiner CE, editors. The Auditory Cortex. New York: Springer-Verlag; 2010. p. 189–208.

119. Snyder RL, Rebscher SJ, Cao KL, et al. Chronic intracochlear electrical stimulation in the neonatally deafened cat. I: expansion of central representation. Hear Res 1990;50:7–33.

120. Shepherd RK, Baxi JH, Hardie NA. Response of inferior colliculus neurons to electrical stimulation of the auditory nerve in neonatally deafened cats. J Neurophysiol 1999;82:1363–80.

121. Friauf E, Kandler K. Auditory projections to the inferior colliculus of the rat are present by birth. Neurosci Lett 1990;120:58–61.

122. Shepherd RK, Javel E. Electrical stimulation of the auditory nerve. I. Correlation of physiological responses with cochlear status. Hear Res 1997;108:112–44.

123. Sly DJ, Heffer LF, White MW, et al. Deafness alters auditory nerve fibre responses to cochlear implant stimulation. Eur J Neurosci 2007;26:510–22.

124. Hancock KE, Noel V, Ryugo DK, et al. Neural coding of interaural time differences with bilateral cochlear implants: effects of congenital deafness. J Neurosci 2010;30:14068–79.

125. Francis HW, Manis PB. Effects of deafferentation on the electrophysiology of ventral cochlear nucleus neurons. Hear Res 2000;149:91–105.

126. Syka J, Popelar J, Kvasnak E, et al. Response properties of neurons in the central nucleus and external and dorsal cortices of the inferior colliculus in guinea pig. Exp Brain Res 2000;133:254–66.

127. Syka J, Rybalko N. Threshold shifts and enhancement of cortical evoked responses after noise exposure in rats. Hear Res 2000;139:59–68.

128. Buras ED, Holt AG, Griffith RD, et al. Changes in glycine immunoreactivity in the rat superior olivary complex following deafness. J Comp Neurol 2006;494: 179–89.

129. Winer JA, Lee CC. The distributed auditory cortex. Hear Res 2007;229:3–13.

130. Kral A, Hartmann R, Tillein J, et al. Congenital auditory deprivation reduces synaptic activity within the auditory cortex in a layer-specific manner. Cereb Cortex 2000;10:714–26.
131. Kral A, Hartmann R, Tillein J, et al. Delayed maturation and sensitive periods in the auditory cortex. Audiol Neurootol 2001;6:346–62.
132. Klinke R, Kral A, Heid S, et al. Recruitment of the auditory cortex in congenitally deaf cats by long-term cochlear electrostimulation. Science 1999;285:1729–33.
133. Ryugo DK, Kretzmer EA, Niparko JK. Restoration of auditory nerve synapses in cats by cochlear implants. Science 2005;310:1490–2.
134. O'Neil JN, Limb CJ, Baker CA. Bilateral effects of unilateral cochlear implantation in congenitally deaf cats. J Comp Neurol 2010;518:2382–404.
135. Eisen MD, Ryugo DK. Hearing molecules: contributions from genetic deafness. Cell Mol Life Sci 2007;64:566–80.

Canine Deafness

George M. Strain, PhD

KEYWORDS

- Sensorineural deafness • Conductive deafness • Pigment-associated deafness
- Hereditary deafness • Presbycusis • Age-related hearing loss
- Noise-induced hearing loss • Ototoxicity

KEY POINTS

- Deafness is common in dogs and has a variety of causes; the most frequent is congenital hereditary sensorineural deafness associated with white pigmentation.
- Conductive deafness often may be resolved, whereas sensorineural deafness is, at present, permanent.
- In addition to hereditary causes of sensorineural deafness, hearing loss can also result from aging (presbycusis), ototoxicity, noise trauma, otitis interna, anesthesia, and several less common causes.
- Because pigment-associated congenital deafness is hereditary, affected animals should not be bred.
- Definitive diagnosis of deafness requires brainstem auditory evoked response testing, because behavioral testing has limited reliability.

INTRODUCTION

Auditory function is important to animals because it is a means by which much of the interaction with its environment occurs; reduction or loss of this function can have a mild or an extreme impact. Deaf animals can survive, but deafness or diminished hearing precludes usefulness in working dogs, diminishes communication in pet-family relationships, impedes communication with conspecifics, and can put affected animals in jeopardy in settings where motor vehicles or predator animals can inflict damage or even death.[1]

Deafness (partial or complete inability to hear) may result from a wide variety of causes. Remedies may exist for some types, but for other types there is no recourse. Knowing an animal's type of deafness is informative in understanding the impact it has on the animal's life, the prognosis for the condition, and any breeding implications.

Funding: N/A.
The author has nothing to disclose.
Department of Comparative Biomedical Sciences, School of Veterinary Medicine, Louisiana State University, Baton Rouge, LA 70803, USA
E-mail address: strain@lsu.edu

Vet Clin Small Anim 42 (2012) 1209–1224
http://dx.doi.org/10.1016/j.cvsm.2012.08.010   **vetsmall.theclinics.com**

This article presents and discusses the types of deafness that may be encountered in clinical practice.

Diagnosis of deafness by behavioral means is often unreliable, because it is difficult to identify unilateral deafness or partial hearing loss by behavioral testing. Dogs able to hear may not respond because of situational anxiety, or may discontinue responding when the stimulus loses interest for them. Deaf dogs may respond because they detect the stimulus through other senses, from visual cues, vibration, or even air movement. Objective diagnosis requires electrodiagnostic testing, usually the brain-stem auditory evoked response (BAER). This is covered in detail elsewhere in this issue and in other references.[2–6]

NORMAL AUDITORY FUNCTION

The frequency range of hearing for dogs is often reported to be 67 Hz to 45 kHz, whereas that of humans, from similar sources, is 64 Hz to 23 kHz.[1] Although comparisons must be made with caution because dissimilar methods of determination have been used, it is clear that dogs detect sounds at much higher frequencies than humans, but differ little on the low frequency end. There is little difference between dogs and humans in detection thresholds for sounds within their optimum frequency range of hearing, in both cases being approximately 0 dB SPL (sound pressure level) over the range of approximately 1 to 10 kHz.[1] Dogs of different sizes from different breeds show little variation in hearing, based on measurements of frequency thresholds and ranges for a single Chihuahua, Dachshund, poodle, and Saint Bernard, where the audiograms were essentially identical.[7] However, the absence of any interbreed differences has not been confirmed through systematic studies.

Successful detection of sound requires patency of the outer and middle ears, and proper function of the middle and internal ears. Identification of the source of a sound requires bilateral hearing, so unilateral deafness impairs this ability. Coverage of normal auditory function is presented in detail elsewhere in this issue and in other sources.[1,8]

Behavioral changes in deaf dogs can be subtle or grossly apparent. Bilaterally deaf puppies often go undetected because they cue off of the behavior of their littermates; they usually are very visually attentive and as a result may seem to have above average intelligence. Unilaterally deaf dogs show difficulty localizing the source of a sound, but often adapt. Hearing loss that is progressive (eg, age-related or from noise trauma) often goes undetected by the owner until a significant level of loss is reached. In hunting or field trial dogs, the distance at which a dog responds to a signal sound decreases. Totally deaf dogs may be more susceptible to being startled, and so should be approached with caution; these dogs should also be protected from undetected dangers, such as motor vehicles. Bilaterally deaf puppies are more challenging to train than hearing puppies, and may be more of a challenge than some owners are willing to accept. Deaf dogs can learn to respond to hand signals and other cues, and function better in households with other dogs whose behavior they can follow.

TYPES OF DEAFNESS

Deafness is not always bilateral, is not always total for an ear, and is not always hereditary. To describe deafness, it is useful to apply pairs of discriminant terms. The discussion next follows that of[9] in explaining the possible presentations of deafness.

Unilateral Versus Bilateral Deafness

Deafness can affect one or both ears. Humans can report unilateral losses, but animals with hearing loss in just one ear are frequently not identified as such unless and until both ears become affected, if the loss is progressive; some are never detected. Unilaterally deaf puppies often exhibit difficulties determining the origin of sounds, which requires bilateral hearing, but often adapt to the condition and no longer show this deficit. Hereditary deafness and hearing loss associated with otitis can be unilateral, whereas ototoxicity (from systemic drug administration), noise-induced hearing loss (NIHL), and age-related hearing loss (ARHL; presbycusis) are typically bilateral.

Partial Versus Total Deafness

If both ears are totally deaf, the animal is obvious in failing to respond to sounds. In litters of puppies this may not be recognized because deaf dogs cue their behavior based on littermates. If hearing loss is partial, the animal may not exhibit any deficit unless it is progressive and until it reaches a level where the dog can no longer cope. This seems acute in onset to the owner when the disease may have been progressing for months or years. Hereditary deafness is usually total in the affected ear, whereas most other types are expressed as partial deafness, at least initially, including NIHL, presbycusis, and ototoxicity.

Syndromic Versus Nonsyndromic Deafness

In many types of deafness in humans, hearing loss is accompanied by disease in other organ systems or abnormalities in phenotype. These include Usher syndrome, where deafness is accompanied by retinitis pigmentosa; Alport syndrome, where nephritis accompanies deafness; and Waardenburg syndrome, where deafness is accompanied by a variety of other disorders, including pigmentation abnormalities. There are no known syndromic types of deafness in dogs. Canine hereditary deafness is usually associated with white skin and hair, but the pigment patterns are not considered to be abnormal and so the deafness is not syndromic.

Peripheral Versus Central Deafness

Deafness can result from retrocochlear (central) disease (cochlear nerve, brainstem, auditory cortex) or from disorders of the peripheral auditory organ and support structures (external ear, middle ear, cochlea). The retrocochlear auditory pathway projects centrally through several brain structures on the way to the thalamus and auditory cortex; at most points in this pathway some auditory fibers ascend ipsilaterally, whereas others decussate and ascend contralaterally. As a result it is difficult for central deafness to result without significant concurrent brain damage that would be reflected by extensive neurologic abnormalities.

TYPES OF PERIPHERAL DEAFNESS

Most cases of deafness in dogs are peripheral, and the rest of this discussion covers types of peripheral deafness. Discriminant pairs of terms are also useful in describing the possible types of peripheral deafness. Peripheral deafness can be sensorineural or conductive, inherited or acquired, or congenital or later onset.

From these pairs of terms, eight possible combinations are theoretically possible. Deafness may be sensorineural, inherited, and congenital, or it may be conductive, acquired, and later onset, and so on.

- Conductive deafness results when sound is reduced or blocked from reaching the internal ear because of outer or middle ear pathologies. Conductive deafness can often be corrected.

- Sensorineural deafness occurs when there is damage to the hair cells or afferent neurons of the cochlea. Sensorineural deafness cannot be corrected at present in mammals, although regeneration of hair cells can occur in avian species.
- Inherited deafness has a genetic basis, whereas acquired deafness does not. At present there are no known hereditary forms of deafness in dogs except those that are congenital, with one possible exception being a condition in Cavalier King Charles spaniels (see later).
- Acquired deafness includes all nonhereditary types of deafness.
- Congenital (literally "with birth") deafness can be hereditary, but is not necessarily so; several other conditions can produce deafness in the perinatal period. Hereditary congenital sensorineural deafness actually does not develop until 3 to 4 weeks of age.
- Deafness that occurs following the perinatal period is later onset.

The types of peripheral deafness that are clinically observed in dogs are summarized in **Table 1**.[9]

Conductive Deafness

Conductive deafness is nearly always acquired and later onset. Ear canal atresia is a rare congenital cause; the ear canal may be delayed in opening or may be permanently sealed. Surgery may be an option. Causes for later-onset conductive deafness include otitis externa and media, middle ear effusion, cerumen impaction, ear canal inflammation from awns or other foreign bodies, middle ear polyps, and possibly otosclerosis, although the last has not been reported in dogs. Some cases of severe and chronic otitis externa require total ear canal ablation and bulla osteotomy; in most cases auditory function is present after the ablation if it was present before surgery.[10] The animal will have conductive deafness from muffling of sounds by the skin over the former ear canal opening, but loud sounds will still be detected.

Table 1
Classifications and examples of different types of peripheral deafness in dogs

	Sensorineural		Conductive	
	Congenital	Later Onset	Congenital	Later Onset
Hereditary	Pigment-associated Non–pigment-associated (Doberman, Puli)	None known	None known	Primary secretory otitis media (Cavalier King Charles spaniel)[a]
Acquired	Perinatal anoxia Dystocia Intrauterine ototoxin exposure	Ototoxin exposure Otitis interna Presbycusis Noise trauma Physical trauma Anesthesia-associated Undetermined	Ear canal atresia	Otitis externa Otitis media Cerumen impaction Ear canal inflammation (awns) Ear canal foreign bodies Middle ear polyps Otosclerosis

[a] Hereditary basis suspected but not confirmed.

From Strain GM. Forms and mechanisms of deafness. In: Deafness in dogs and cats. Wallingford (UK): CAB International; 2011. p. 45; with permission.

A condition called primary secretory otitis media (or glue ear, or otitis media with effusion) is a later-onset form of conductive deafness discussed in more detail elsewhere in this issue. Because the condition occurs primarily in the Cavalier King Charles spaniel breed (although it has been reported once each in a Dachshund, boxer, and Shih Tzû),[11] there may be a hereditary basis for the disorder. It has also been suggested that the condition may be the result of pharyngeal conformation, resulting from a thick soft palate and reduced nasopharyngeal aperture.[12]

Sensorineural Deafness

The sound-detecting structures of the internal ear, the cochlea and its organ of Corti, contain two targets through which pathology may produce sensorineural deafness: the hair cells and the stria vascularis (**Fig. 1**). The organ of Corti has one row of inner hair cells, which are the primary transduction cells for audition, and three rows of outer hair cells, which actively amplify sound. Loss of cochlear hair cells produces deafness. The stria vascularis, a modified vascular structure on the outer wall of the cochlear duct, is responsible for maintaining high potassium levels in the endolymph fluid that surrounds the stereocilia of the hair cells. Damage to the stria vascularis, or the absence of functioning melanocytes in the stria, results in secondary loss of hair cells and deafness. Melanocytes in the stria play a critical role in potassium level maintenance in the endolymph.[13] The most frequent clinical presentation of sensorineural deafness is congenital hereditary deafness, followed by presbycusis, then ototoxicity and noise trauma, then anesthesia-associated deafness.

Internal ear abnormalities, hereditary or from developmental anomalies, have been classified into three types[14,15]: (1) morphogenetic, (2) neuroepithelial, and (3) cochleosaccular or Scheibe-type. Morphogenetic abnormalities include structural deformities

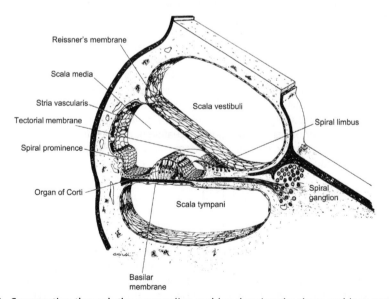

Fig. 1. Cross-section through the mammalian cochlea showing the three cochlear compartments (the scala vestibuli, the scala tympani, and between them the cochlear duct or scala media); the organ of Corti; the spiral ganglion; and the stria vascularis. Hair cells in the organ of Corti and the stria vascularis are the targets of processes causing sensorineural deafness. (*Courtesy of* Don W. Fawcett, MD.)

of either the bony or membranous labyrinths that result from mutations acting in early development of these structures. Semicircular canals may be absent, and the cochlear duct may be reduced or even absent. Because of the severity of the abnormalities the deafness is not easily classifiable as either sensorineural or conductive. These are rare.

Neuroepithelial abnormalities appear at the end of cochlear development (3–4 weeks after birth in dogs) and result from hair cell degeneration that occurs after the normal pattern of development. The stria vascularis and Reissner membrane are normal until late stages in the degenerative process. Vestibular dysfunction may be a component, deafness is complete, and both ears seem to be symmetrically affected. This type occurs in the Doberman pinscher and perhaps in the few other breeds with hereditary congenital deafness that is not pigment-associated. The mechanisms for this type of deafness are not known in dogs, but in humans and mouse models the causes are frequently channelopathies: mutations in genes responsible for neuron membrane ion channels, especially potassium ion channels.[16]

Cochleo-saccular or Scheibe-type abnormalities also occur late in cochlear development, but deafness results from initial degeneration of the stria vascularis. Strial degeneration results in loss of the elevated potassium concentration in the endolymph, and the hair cells degenerate, Reissner membrane collapses, and other cochlear structures eventually collapse and degenerate, including spiral ganglion cells whose axons form the cochlear branch of the eighth cranial nerve. In some species the saccule of the vestibular system may also degenerate, but it is not clear how often this occurs in affected dogs. Deafness may be unilateral or bilateral, and is total in an affected ear, although in rare cases hearing for the very high frequencies may be retained but at frequencies so high as to be of limited use in daily life. This retained hearing may reflect the continuity of the fluids between the cochlear duct and the vestibular organs, and the location in the cochlea for normal high-frequency hearing at its base; the degeneration of the stria vascularis in the cochlea and loss of high potassium levels around the hair cell stereocilia may be compensated for by vestibular endolymph. Most occurrences of cochleo-saccular deafness are associated with the genes responsible for white or lightened pigmentation in skin and hair (piebald or merle in the dog) where the genes suppress melanocyte function to produce white. Suppression of melanocytes in the stria vascularis by these genes disrupts their regulation of the endolymph composition, and deafness ensues as a secondary effect. Pigment-associated deafness is the most common type of deafness in dogs and cats, and is by far the most common form of congenital deafness.

Sensorineural deafness can also result from neuroepithelial and cochleo-saccular cochlear degeneration that is a result of nongenetic causes.

Hereditary Deafness

Pigment-associated deafness
Most hereditary deafness in dogs is pigment-associated, of the cochleo-saccular pathology type, and is specifically associated with either the recessive alleles of the piebald gene (S) or the dominant allele of the merle (M) gene. Dog breeds with reported congenital deafness number more than 90 (**Box 1**). Congenital deafness is not necessarily hereditary, but there is good evidence for a genetic basis in many breeds, especially those with white or dilute pigmentation patterns. In recent years, significant effort has gone into documenting the prevalence of deafness in breeds affected by pigment-associated deafness[17–23]; rates vary by breed, ranging from a high of 30% (unilateral and bilateral) in Dalmatians in the United States, to 1.3% in colored bull terriers.[18] Hearing testing of puppies can be performed beginning at about 5 weeks of age;

Box 1
Dog breeds with reported congenital deafness. Dogs of any breed can be affected from a variety of causes, but breeds with white pigmentation are most often affected

Akita	Dalmatian	Old English Sheepdog
American bulldog	Dappled Dachshund	Papillon
American-Canadian shepherd	Doberman pinscher	Perro de Carea Leonés
American Eskimo	Dogo Argentino	Pit bull terrier
American hairless terrier	English bulldog	Pointer/English pointer
American Staffordshire terrier	English cocker spaniel	Presa Canario
Anatolian shepherd	English setter	Puli
Australian cattle dog	Foxhound	Rhodesian ridgeback
Australian shepherd	Fox terrier	Rat terrier
Beagle	French bulldog	Rottweiler
Belgian sheepdog/	German shepherd	Saint Bernard
Groenendael		
Belgian Tervuren	German shorthaired pointer	Samoyed
Bichon Frise	Great Dane	Schnauzer
Border collie	Great Pyrenees	Scottish terrier
Borzoi	Greyhound	Sealyham terrier
Boston terrier	Havanese	Shetland sheepdog
Boxer	Ibizan hound	Shih Tzû
Brittney spaniel	Icelandic sheepdog	Shropshire terrier
Bulldog	Italian greyhound	Siberian husky
Bull terrier	Jack/Parson Russell terrier	Soft coated Wheaten terrier
Canaan dog	Japanese Chin	Springer spaniel
Cardigan Welsh Corgi	Kuvasz	Sussex spaniel
Catahoula leopard dog	Labrador retriever	Tibetan spaniel
Catalan shepherd	Löwchen	Tibetan terrier
Cavalier King Charles spaniel	Maltese	Toy fox terrier
Chihuahua	Miniature pinscher	Toy poodle
Chinese crested	Miniature poodle	Walker American foxhound
Chow chow	Mongrel	West Highland white terrier
Cocker spaniel	Newfoundland Landseer	Whippet
Collie	Norwegian Dunkerhound	Yorkshire terrier
Coton de Tulear	Nova Scotia duck tolling retriever	

From Strain GM. Deafness in dogs and cats. Available at: http://www.lsu.edu/deafness/deaf.htm

---

breeders in breeds with significant deafness prevalence rates frequently have BAER testing performed before placing puppies and may cull bilaterally deaf puppies.

The piebald and merle genes suppress melanocytes, producing white or dilution of pigmentation in skin and hair, blue irises in some dogs, and disrupted function in the stria vascularis, resulting in deafness. Significant associations between the absence of iris pigment and deafness have been shown for several breeds with the piebald gene, including Dalmatian, English setter, and English cocker spaniel.[18]

Piebald

The *S* locus has four alleles. The dominant allele *S* (for self) produces solid color. Three recessive alleles express increasing white in the coat: Irish spotting (s^i), piebald (s^p), and extreme white piebald (s^w). Examples of breeds carrying these alleles are as follows: Irish spotting, Basenji and Bernese mountain dog; piebald, English springer spaniel, fox terrier, and beagle; and extreme white piebald, Dalmatian, bull terrier, and Samoyed. Breeds may contain within their population two or even three of the different recessive alleles[24]; the identification of which alleles are present in a breed is often uncertain because there are no genetic markers to distinguish them.

Merle

The *M* locus has two alleles: the recessive allele *m* produces uniform pigmentation, whereas the dominant allele *M*, known as merle or dapple, produces a random pattern of diluted pigmentation overlying uniform pigmentation; it also increases the amount of white spotting on the coat. Dogs homozygous for the dominant allele can be deaf and frequently have ocular abnormalities; even heterozygous dogs can be deaf, but there may be breed differences in the prevalence of deafness in merle carriers.[20] Breeds carrying the merle allele include Shetland sheepdog, Australian shepherd, Cardigan Welsh Corgi, and Dachshund. In general, the prevalence of deafness in dogs carrying merle is similar to that of breeds with piebald. Some breeds carry merle and piebald, and some breeds (eg, Great Danes) with merle also carry a modifier gene known as harlequin.[25]

Gene identification: merle

The merle gene has been sequenced, and has been identified to be a mutation in the dominant allele of the *SILV* pigmentation gene, located on canine chromosome 10 (CFA10, **Table 2**).[26] The mutation is a 253 base pair short interspersed element located just before exon 11 in the gene, and includes a multiple adenine repeat (poly-A) tail that must be 90 to 100 adenine repeats in length to cause expression of the merle phenotype. The identification of the gene has not yet provided an explanation of the basis for the deafness associated with its presence in a dog. A locus for the harlequin gene, which modifies expression of merle so that diluted areas become white, has been reported on canine chromosome 9 (CFA9, see **Table 2**).[27] It is not known whether harlequin has any association with deafness; Great Danes can carry merle, harlequin, and piebald.

Gene identification: piebald

The various alleles of *S* have been reported to be mutations of the microphthalmia-associated transcription factor (*MITF*) gene, located on canine chromosome 20 (CFA20, see **Table 2**).[28] Two mutations were identified in a 3.5-kb region upstream of the M promoter region, that in various combinations were said to generate the different alleles: a short interspersed element insertion present in piebald and extreme white piebald breeds but missing in Irish spotting and solid breeds, and a polymorphism in the promoter region of the gene present in solid dogs. A separate research group was unable to duplicate all of the study's reported findings[29] and a third is pursuing a relationship between Irish spotting and the gene *KITLG* (c-Kit ligand) on canine chromosome 15 (CFA15, see **Table 2**).[30] *KITLG* plays a role in melanogenesis. As with the merle gene, no studies of these genes have provided an explanation for the associated deafness.

Inheritance of pigment-associated deafness

The inheritance of pigment-associated deafness seems complex and does not parallel the inheritance of the associated pigment genes merle (simple dominant) and piebald (simple recessive). Numerous studies have attempted to identify the mechanism of inheritance of deafness using either a statistical technique called complex segregation analysis of pedigrees or microsatellite marker studies of DNA from affected dogs, without a consensus[21,31–36]; most proposed some version of an autosomal-recessive mechanism, but not one that is simple mendelian autosomal-recessive. A recent study of deafness in Australian stumpy-tail cattle dogs used a whole genome screen of microsatellite markers and identified a locus on canine chromosome 10 that was significantly linked to deafness.[21] Located within that locus is the gene

Table 2
Genes implicated in pigment-associated hereditary sensorineural deafness in dogs

Common Name	Chromosome	Gene Name	Gene Product/Function	Mutation
Merle (*M*)	CFA10	*SILV*	Melanocyte protein Pmel17; plays a role in pigmentation patterns	A 256 bp retrotransposon insertion with a poly-A tail
Piebald (*S*)	CFA20	*MITF* (microphthalmia-associated transcription factor)	Regulates *SILV* and the gene *tyrosinase*, involved in melanin synthesis and melanocyte development	Two mutations upstream of the M promoter region of the gene; different combinations result in the different recessive alleles of *S*
Piebald – Irish spotting (*s^i*)	CFA15	*KITLG* (c-Kit ligand)	Plays a role in melanogenesis; possible origin of the Irish spotting allele of *S*	Unknown
Harlequin	CFA9	Unknown	Modifies the effects of *M*; produces complete hypopigmentation of areas otherwise white in merles	Unknown
None	CFA10	Possibly *SOX10*	Transcription factor that regulates *MITF* Possible deafness gene in Australian stumpy-tailed cattle dogs	Unknown

SOX10, a homeobox gene that is an activator of the gene *MITF*. However, sequencing of *SOX10* in several affected dogs showed no mutations, and the study has not been repeated in dogs from other affected breeds, so it is not yet clear that a mutation of *SOX10* is causative.

At present, genes located on canine chromosomes 9, 10, 15, and 20 have been investigated that play a role in pigmentation in the dog and that may play a role in deafness (see **Table 2**); many more genes have been identified to be involved in pigmentation and linked to different forms of deafness in humans and in mouse mutations.[37] Much work remains to solve the genetic basis of this form of deafness. Until DNA-based tests become available to identify dogs carrying gene mutations responsible for hereditary deafness, affected dogs should not be bred, even those deaf in just one ear.

Doberman pinscher

Bilateral congenital deafness accompanied by vestibular disease in Doberman pinschers has a neuroepithelial cochlear pathology and has an autosomal-recessive mode of inheritance based on pedigree analysis.[38] Vestibular signs of head tilt, ataxia, and circling behavior develop between birth and 12 weeks of age, but the animals adapt to them with time; the deafness is permanent. Similar presentations have been reported in beagle, Akita, and possibly in Tibetan and Shropshire terriers.[25] No gene linked to the disorder has been reported, and the mechanisms responsible for the cochlear and vestibular hair cell degeneration are unknown.

Pointers

A champion field trial pointer bitch reputed to have experienced a nervous breakdown was used as foundation breeding stock to develop a line of dogs with enhanced anxious behavior to support research in human anxiety disorders.[39] Concurrent with the breeding for increased anxious behavior was the appearance of deafness in affected dogs. Most anxious dogs were bilaterally deaf by 3 months of age, but not all were affected, suggesting incomplete penetrance; the cochlear degeneration is of the neuroepithelial type.[40] Pedigree analysis suggested autosomal-recessive inheritance, but because of tight inbreeding, other mechanisms of inheritance could not be ruled out.[39] Responsible genes and mechanisms have not been identified. Deafness does not seem to develop in pointers unrelated to this special-bred kindred.

Presbycusis

Presbycusis, or ARHL, is primarily sensorineural but may also include conductive hearing loss and central changes. It is progressive, usually bilaterally symmetric, and generally affects high frequencies before low frequencies. In humans it may be accompanied by tinnitus and has no known treatment or cure. The deficits can be exacerbated by NIHL, hypertension, and diabetes. Human males are affected more than females, but it is unclear if this holds true for dogs. The primary mechanism is degeneration of the stria vascularis,[41] but concurrent degeneration of the organ of Corti and ganglion cells is observed. Genetic factors are important in human ARHL, but no studies have examined genetic effects in dogs.

A 7-year study documented tone burst-derived BAER thresholds in middle-sized dogs as presbycusis developed.[42] Hearing thresholds began to increase at 8 to 10 years of age, and the mid- to high-range frequencies of 8 to 32 kHz were affected first. The loss was progressive and expanded to cover the entire frequency range. Life expectancies vary in dogs based on body size, with small breed dogs living longer than large breed dogs, so the age of onset of ARHL likely differs between large and small breeds. The pattern of pathologies seen in geriatric dogs with ARHL included reductions in the stria vascularis, numbers of hair cells, and numbers of spiral ganglion cells,[43] mirroring human pathology.

Ototoxicity

Many drugs and chemicals have been identified that are toxic to the internal ear, both the cochlea and the vestibular organs. More than 180 compounds and classes of compounds have been identified as ototoxic.[44] Some produce effects that are reversible if detected early, such as the salicylates, but most produce effects that are permanent by the time of discovery. Effects can be auditory or vestibular or both, unilateral or bilateral, and may result in partial or total functional loss. Toxicity may result from parenteral or topical application, and can result from long-term and acute exposures. Synergism may result from concurrent ototoxic drug exposure with presbycusis or noise trauma. Mechanisms of toxicity may be through direct damage of hair cells (neuroepithelial) or indirect effects through damage to the stria vascularis (cochleo-saccular).

Ototoxic drugs and chemicals can be classified into broad groups: antibiotics (aminoglycosides and others); loop diuretics; antiseptics; antineoplastic agents; and miscellaneous agents. The drug most frequently associated with ototoxicity is the aminoglycoside gentamicin, which can also be nephrotoxic. Despite the known potential toxicity of gentamicin, it is still probably the most commonly used antibiotic for topical treatment of otitis externa, in part because of its high efficacy, broad spectrum of gram-negative activity, and low cost. Its toxicity is unpredictable and does not seem to reliably be related to dose, frequency, or route of administration.[45] The mechanism of toxicity is a sequence of iron chelation, followed by free radical formation, and then caspase-dependent apoptosis.[46] Although drug manufacturers may state that gentamicin-induced ototoxicity can be reversible, this has not been the author's experience.

Human studies have shown that coadministration of aspirin or other antioxidants during dialysis prevents or reduces gentamicin ototoxicity,[47] but it is not known whether postdeafness treatment has any value in restoring hearing loss. Ototoxicity is covered in more detail elsewhere in this issue.

Noise-Induced Hearing Loss

NIHL, or noise trauma, increasingly affects humans and animals. Military dogs exposed to loud percussive sounds, hunting companion dogs (especially Labrador retrievers), dogs housed in kennels with high ambient noise levels,[48,49] and even dogs shipped by airplane in cargo compartments where there are high ambient noise levels may all develop NIHL.[44] Protective reflexes exist where middle ear muscles contract in response to loud sounds to reduce sound levels reaching the inner ear, but the reflexes are too slow for percussive sounds, such as gunfire, and only provide limited protection against very loud noises. Hearing loss is primarily caused by loss of hair cells from mechanical disruption, but extreme sounds can also damage the tympanum and ossicles. NIHL is a cumulative process where sound intensity and duration of exposure determine the damage. The US Occupational Safety and Health Administration and federal agencies in other countries have established regulations for permissible workplace noise exposures for people.[50] Separate standards have not been developed for dogs, but human standards provide reasonable criteria unless future studies suggest more sensitive standards. It should be noted that Occupational Safety and Health Administration standards refer to continuous noise exposure; percussive sounds have the potential to produce significant damage, so efforts should be used to protect the hearing of hunting dogs exposed to gunfire and military dogs exposed to explosions, just as hunters protect their own hearing with protective devices. However, effective devices for noise protection are not yet commercially available for dogs.

Noise exposure can produce temporary and permanent hearing loss. Gradual recovery may occur with some exposures if they are brief; this type of loss is called a temporary threshold shift. Repeated or continued exposures result in permanent hearing loss, or permanent threshold shift. NIHL is greater in older subjects, and there seem to be genetic differences in susceptibility, including increased sensitivity in subjects with white pigmentation.[51] Damage is produced in the organ of Corti, stria vascularis, spiral ganglion cells, and spiral ligament. Temporary threshold shift is associated with effects on the stria vascularis, whereas permanent threshold shifts are associated with damage to hair cells in the organ of Corti,[51] including disruption of stereocilia and the cuticular plate (their attachment point to the hair cell body), generation of reactive oxygen species, apoptosis, and necrosis.

Dogs seem to be more often affected than cats, perhaps simply because of greater opportunities for exposure. Associated behavior is a gradual reduction in the distance at which a dog responds to a voice or whistle command. The hearing loss is gradual and cumulative, so owners often report an apparent acute onset even though the dog was undergoing progressive damage. Animals adapt to the loss until a point is reached where they can no longer compensate. NIHL often is accompanied by ARHL, and in humans there can also be the presence of tinnitus. Studies have shown that concurrent administration of antioxidants, such as N-acetylcysteine, have protectant effects, and some agents, such as adenosine A_1 receptor agonists, may even be effective postexposure.[52]

Anesthesia-Associated Deafness

Although uncommon, some dogs or cats that undergo anesthesia, especially for dental cleaning procedures, recover from anesthesia with bilateral deafness that in most cases is permanent.[53] In a study of 62 reported cases in dogs and cats, no association was observed between deafness and breed, gender, anesthetic drug used, or dog size.[53] Forty-three of the reported cases occurred after dental procedures, and 16 cases after ear cleanings. Geriatric animals seemed more susceptible to the hearing loss, which might reflect a bias because of dental procedures being performed more often on older animals. In at least one case, deafness was the result of a persistent otitis media with effusion, suggesting possible eustachian tube dysfunction subsequent to vigorous jaw manipulation during a dental procedure (unpublished observation). For most cases the cause is unknown and ongoing studies are pursuing possible mechanisms.

Otitis Interna-Associated Deafness

Infections that reach the internal ear have the potential to produce sensorineural deafness, and are frequently accompanied by vestibular signs because of connections between the fluid-filled compartments of the cochlea and vestibular organs. Otitis interna is common, and usually results from extension of otitis media. Factors that influence or determine whether an infection results in permanent deafness have not been identified, but the duration of the infection may be a factor. The appearance of vestibular signs that suggest otitis interna should suggest immediate initiation of appropriate diagnostic tests to determine the cause of the signs, and if they are related to an infectious otitis antimicrobial therapy should be instituted to minimize the potential for hearing loss.

OTHER HEARING CONDITIONS
Tinnitus

Tinnitus is the perception of sounds in the absence of actual external sounds.[54] Objective tinnitus is the perception of actual sounds generated by the ear, from turbulent blood flow near the cochlea or abnormalities in the muscles near the ear or eustachian tube, and in rare cases generated by the cochlea itself. They are low in intensity, but can be heard by others when in close proximity or by means of a stethoscope. Objective tinnitus has been reported in dogs and cats, usually as a high frequency tone that does not seem to bother the animal. Subjective tinnitus (ringing in the ears) is the perception of phantom sounds when no actual sound is present; this is the form typically meant when tinnitus is used as a term without a modifier.

In humans, subjective tinnitus exhibits with variable features that can be so severe as to be disabling. It may seem to originate in one or both ears or seem to originate in the center of the head; may be continuous or intermittent; and may be perceived as a single or multiple pure tones or any number of various other sounds that include hissing, roaring, whistling, chirping, clicking, and buzzing. Tinnitus most often results from exposure to loud noises, especially gunfire or loud music, or presbycusis, and less often from ototoxic drugs, meningitis, encephalitis, stroke, and traumatic brain injury.

Because subjective tinnitus is subjective, it is not possible to know if dogs experience it. Some dogs with an acute onset of deafness exhibit anxious behavior that may indicate tinnitus, but may instead just reflect a response to the loss of hearing. The behavior is typically short lived, suggesting that the dogs adapt if it is indeed a continuing sensation.

Hyperacusis

Increased sensitivity to sounds that otherwise would not be bothersome is called hyperacusis. It can result from peripheral auditory disorders, central nervous system disorders, and hormonal and infectious disorders, but the cause is often unknown.[55] Noise-induced hearing loss and facial nerve damage are common origins. Hyperacusis often accompanies tinnitus and can precede its appearance. Some dog owners report an apparent hypersensitivity to sound, but BAER results have been normal. There have been no studies of this condition in dogs or cats.

Otoacoustic Emissions

Although not a hearing disorder, the ear can generate sounds (otoacoustic emissions [OAE]), either spontaneously or in response to introduced sounds. OAE are thought to reflect the function of outer hair cells of the cochlea, which contain contractile proteins that allow the cells to shorten or lengthen at a rapid frequency.[56] Spontaneous OAE are present in most normal ears at very low levels, and can occasionally be loud enough to be detected by the unaided listener.[57] Evoked OAE provide a sensitive early indicator of loss of auditory function. Evoked OAE are used clinically to assess auditory function in humans,[56] and have begun to be reported for deafness screening applications in dogs.[58] Two types of evoked OAE are in use: transient evoked OAE and distortion product OAE.[56] OAE are discussed in more detail elsewhere in this issue.

SUMMARY

Deafness is common in dogs and has a variety of causes. The most frequent is congenital hereditary sensorineural deafness associated with white pigmentation.

Conductive deafness often may be resolved, whereas sensorineural deafness is, at present, permanent. However, it has recently been demonstrated that hair cells can be generated from mouse stem cells in culture,[59] so therapies may become available in the future. In addition to hereditary causes of sensorineural deafness, hearing loss can also result from aging (presbycusis), ototoxicity, noise trauma, otitis interna, anesthesia, and several less common causes. Because pigment-associated congenital deafness is hereditary, affected animals should not be bred. Definitive diagnosis of deafness requires BAER testing, because behavioral testing has limited reliability.

REFERENCES

1. Strain GM. Physiology of the auditory system. In: Deafness in dogs and cats. Wallingford (UK): CAB International; 2011. p. 23–39.
2. Wilson WJ, Mills PC. Brainstem auditory-evoked responses in dogs. Am J Vet Res 2005;66:2177–87.
3. Strain GM. Brainstem auditory evoked response (BAER). In: Deafness in dogs and cats. Wallingford (UK): CAB International; 2011. p. 83–107.
4. Strain GM. Other tests of auditory function. In: Deafness in dogs and cats. Wallingford (UK): CAB International; 2011. p. 108–16.
5. Strain GM, Green KD, Twedt AC, et al. Brain stem auditory evoked potentials from bone stimulation in dogs. Am J Vet Res 1993;54:1817–21.
6. Strain GM, Tedford BL, Jackson RM. Postnatal development of the brainstem auditory-evoked potential in dogs. Am J Vet Res 1991;52:410–5.
7. Heffner HE. Hearing in large and small dogs: absolute thresholds and size of the tympanic membrane. Behav Neurosci 1983;97:310–8.
8. Jahn AF, Santos-Sacchi J. Physiology of the ear. 2nd edition. San Diego: Singular Publishing Group; 2001.
9. Strain GM. Forms and mechanisms of deafness. In: Deafness in dogs and cats. Wallingford (UK): CAB International; 2011. p. 40–52.
10. Krahwinkel DJ, Pardo AD, Sims MH, et al. Effect of total ablation of the external acoustic meatus and bulla osteotomy on auditory function in dogs. J Am Vet Med Assoc 1993;202:949–52.
11. Stern-Bertholtz W, Sjöström L, Hårkanson NW. Primary secretory otitis media in the Cavalier King Charles spaniel: a review of 61 cases. J Small Anim Pract 2003;44:253–6.
12. Hayes GM, Friend EJ, Jeffery ND. Relationship between pharyngeal conformation and otitis media with effusion in Cavalier King Charles spaniels. Vet Rec 2010;167:55–8.
13. Steel KP, Barkway C. Another role for melanocytes: their importance for normal stria vascularis development in the mammalian inner ear. Development 1989; 107:453–63.
14. Steel KP, Bock GR. Hereditary inner-ear abnormalities in animals. Arch Otolaryngol 1986;109:22–9.
15. Steel KP. Inherited hearing defects in mice. Annu Rev Genet 1995;29:675–701.
16. Lv P, Wei D, Yamoah EN. K_v7-type channel currents in spiral ganglion neurons. Involvement in sensorineural hearing loss. J Biol Chem 2010;285:34699–707.
17. Strain GM, Kearney MT, Gignac IJ, et al. Brainstem auditory evoked potential assessment of congenital deafness in Dalmatians: associations with phenotypic markers. J Vet Intern Med 1992;6:175–82.
18. Strain GM. Deafness prevalence and pigmentation and gender associations in dog breeds at risk. Vet J 2004;167:23–32.

19. Platt S, Freeman J, di Stefani A, et al. Prevalence of unilateral and bilateral deafness in border collies and association with phenotype. J Vet Intern Med 2006;20: 1355–62.

20. Strain GM, Clark LA, Wahl JM, et al. Prevalence of deafness in dogs heterozygous and homozygous for the merle allele. J Vet Intern Med 2009;23:282–6.

21. Sommerlad S, McRae AF, McDonald B, et al. Congenital sensorineural deafness in Australian stumpy-tail cattle dogs is an autosomal recessive trait that maps to CFA10. PLoS One 2010;5:e13364.

22. De Risio L, Lewis T, Freeman J, et al. Prevalence, heritability and genetic correlations of congenital sensorineural deafness and pigmentation phenotypes in the Border Collie. Vet J 2011;188:286–90.

23. Comito B, Knowles KE, Strain GM. Congenital deafness in Jack Russell terriers: prevalence and association with phenotype. Vet J 2012;193:404–7.

24. Little CC. The inheritance of coat color in dogs. New York: Howell Book House; 1957. p. 194.

25. Strain GM. Hereditary deafness. In: Deafness in dogs and cats. Wallingford (UK): CAB International; 2011. p. 53–69.

26. Clark LA, Wahl JM, Rees CA, et al. Retrotransposon insertion in SILV is responsible for merle patterning of the domestic dog. Proc Natl Acad Sci U S A 2006; 103:1376–81.

27. Clark LA, Starr AN, Tsai KL, et al. Genome-wide linkage scan localizes the harlequin locus in the Great Dane to chromosome 9. Gene 2008;418:49–52.

28. Karlsson EK, Baranowska I, Wade CM, et al. Efficient mapping of mendelian traits in dogs through genome-wide association. Nat Genet 2007;39:1321–8.

29. Schmutz SM, Berryere TG, Dreger DL. MITF and white spotting in dogs: a population study. J Hered 2009;100:S66–74.

30. Starr AN, Tsai KL, Noorai RE, et al. Investigation of KITLG as a candidate gene for Irish spotting in dogs. In: Fyfe J, Murphy W, Ostrander E, et al, editors. Proceedings of the 5th International Conference on Advances in Canine and Feline Genomics and Inherited Diseases. Baltimore (MD); 2010.

31. Famula TR, Oberbauer AM, Sousa CA. Complex segregation analysis of deafness in Dalmatians. Am J Vet Res 2000;61:550–3.

32. Muhle AC, Jaggy A, Stricker C, et al. Further contributions to the genetic aspect of congenital sensorineural deafness in Dalmatians. Vet J 2002;163:311–8.

33. Juraschko K, Meyer-Lindenberg A, Nolte I, et al. A regressive model analysis of congenital sensorineural deafness in German Dalmatian dogs. Mamm Genome 2003;14:547–54.

34. Cargill EJ, Famula TR, Strain GM, et al. Heritability and segregation analysis of deafness in U.S. Dalmatians. Genetics 2004;166:1385–93.

35. Famula TR, Cargill EG, Strain GM. Heritability and complex segregation analysis of deafness in Jack Russell terriers. BMC Vet Res 2007;3:31.

36. Strain GM. White noise: pigment-associated deafness. Vet J 2011;188:247–9.

37. Van Camp G, Smith RJH. Hereditary Hearing Loss Homepage. Available at: http://hereditaryhearingloss.org. Accessed June 1, 2012.

38. Wilkes MK, Palmer AC. Congenital deafness and vestibular deficit in the Doberman. J Small Anim Pract 1992;33:218–24.

39. Steinberg SA, Klein E, Killens RL, et al. Inherited deafness among nervous pointer dogs. J Hered 1994;85:56–9.

40. Coppens AG, Gilbert-Gregory S, Steinberg SA, et al. Inner ear histopathology in "nervous pointer dogs" with severe hearing loss. Hear Res 2005;200:51–62.

41. Liu XZ, Yan D. Aging and hearing loss. J Pathol 2007;211:188–97.

42. Ter Haar G, Venker-van Haagen AJ, van den Brom WE, et al. Effects of aging on brainstem responses to toneburst auditory stimuli: a cross-sectional and longitudinal study in dogs. J Vet Intern Med 2008;22:937–45.

43. Ter Haar G, de Groot JC, Venker-van Haagen AJ, et al. Effects of aging on inner ear morphology in dogs in relation to brainstem responses to toneburst auditory stimuli. J Vet Intern Med 2009;23:536–43.

44. Strain GM. Later onset deafness. In: Deafness in dogs and cats. Wallingford (UK): CAB International; 2011. p. 70–82.

45. Strain GM, Merchant SR, Neer TM, et al. Ototoxicity assessment of a gentamicin sulfate otic preparation in dogs. Am J Vet Res 1995;56:532–8.

46. Rizzi MD, Hirose K. Aminoglycoside ototoxicity. Curr Opin Otolaryngol Head Neck Surg 2007;15:352–7.

47. Chen Y, Huang WG, Zha DJ, et al. Aspirin attenuates gentamicin ototoxicity: from the laboratory to the clinic. Hear Res 2007;226:178–82.

48. Coppola CL, Enns RM, Grandin T. Noise in the animal shelter environment: building design and the effects of daily noise exposure. J Appl Anim Welf Sci 2006;9:1–7.

49. Scheifele P, Martin D, Clark JG, et al. Effect of kennel noise on hearing in dogs. Am J Vet Res 2012;73:482–9.

50. OSHA. Proposed occupational noise exposure regulation. Fed Regist 1974;39: 37773–84.

51. Ohlemiller KK. Recent findings and emerging questions in cochlear noise injury. Hear Res 2008;245:5–17.

52. Wong AC, Guo CX, Gupta R, et al. Post exposure administration of A_1 adenosine receptor agonists attenuates noise-induced hearing loss. Hear Res 2010;260: 81–8.

53. Stevens-Sparks CK, Strain GM. Post-anesthesia deafness in dogs and cats following dental and otic procedures. Vet Anaesth Analg 2010;37:347–51.

54. Møller AR. Tinnitus: presence and future. In: Langguth B, Hajak G, Kleinjung T, et al, editors. Progress in brain research, vol. 166. Amsterdam: Elsevier; 2007. p. 3–16.

55. Katzenell U, Segal S. Hyperacusis: review and clinical guidelines. Otol Neurotol 2001;22:321–7.

56. Hall JW. Handbook of otoacoustic emissions. Clifton Park (NY): Delmar; 2000. p. 635.

57. Ruggero MA, Kramek B, Rich NC. Spontaneous otoacoustic emissions in a dog. Hear Res 1984;13:293–6.

58. McBrearty A, Penderis J. Transient evoked otoacoustic emissions testing for screening of sensorineural deafness in puppies. J Vet Intern Med 2011;25: 1366–71.

59. Oshima K, Shin K, Diensthuber M, et al. Mechanosensitive hair cell-like cells from embryonic and induced pluripotent stem cells. Cell 2010;141:704–16.

Canine Hearing Loss Management

Lesa Scheifele[a], John Greer Clark, PhD[b],*,
Peter M. Scheifele, PhD[c,d]

KEYWORDS

- Hearing loss management • Canine hearing loss • Sign language • Vibrotactile
- Hearing loss prevention • Hearing aid amplification

KEY POINTS

- Consider whether canine hearing loss has social and emotional parallels to human hearing loss.

Regardless of whether these parallels exist, we must also consider the following:

- If hearing loss has a direct impact on owner's interactions with the hearing-impaired dog and how communication can be enhanced.
- Whether any safety concerns might arise for the animal or its humans because of diminished hearing.
- And whether there are any recommendations that the veterinarian might share with the dog owner or handler to help mitigate the impact of any existing hearing loss.

INTRODUCTION

Is it possible that dog owners project their fears of personal hearing loss onto their pets? The thought of developing a hearing loss is indeed frightening for many people. Helen Keller, who was both deaf and blind, once noted that her loss of hearing was far more disconcerting than her loss of sight. As she stated, her blindness separated her from the things in her life that she enjoyed, but it was her hearing loss that separated her from the people in her life that she loved.

Very quickly after a dog enters one's home, either as a family pet (or dare we say family member) or as a working partner, a close bond develops in which the owner/handler wishes only the best for his or her companion. When this loved animal develops a hearing loss, or is suspected to have and subsequently confirmed to have a congenital deafness, it is only natural for owners to project onto their canine companion their

The authors have nothing to disclose.
[a] The Lost Ark, 3104 Ninnichuck Road, Bethel, OH 45106, USA; [b] Department of Communication Sciences and Disorders, University of Cincinnati, 3202 Eden Avenue, Room 344, Cincinnati, OH 45267, USA; [c] Department of Communication Sciences and Disorders, University of Cincinnati, 3202 Eden Avenue Room 344, Cincinnati, OH 45267, USA; [d] Department of Medical Education, University of Cincinnati, 3202 Eden Avenue Room 344, Cincinnati, OH 45267, USA
* Corresponding author.
E-mail address: jg.clark@uc.edu

Vet Clin Small Anim 42 (2012) 1225–1239
http://dx.doi.org/10.1016/j.cvsm.2012.08.009
0195-5616/12/$ – see front matter © 2012 Elsevier Inc. All rights reserved.

own fears of hearing loss and the perceived impact such loss would have on the life of the dog.

Importance of the Sense of Hearing versus the Sense of Smell

As we discuss the impact of hearing loss on dogs, we need to keep in mind that dogs rely on their sense of smell more heavily than their sense of hearing. Humans have about 6 million receptors for scent, whereas dogs, depending on breed, can have up to 300 million![1]

Whereas humans often judge on appearance, dogs assess by scent.[2] Not only can they identify a stranger by scent, but they can smell if a new dog acquaintance is male or female, mature or not, if a female is ready to breed, if she is nursing pups, if there is a health problem, and some of the animal's mood. From a human perspective it might be somewhat disconcerting if everyone met on the street could tell that much about us by just being nearby.

A dog's daily life would be affected much more by the loss of smell than by the loss of hearing. Dogs follow scent trails to find potential prey (as anyone who has had to chase a beagle through dark woods is sorely aware), find their toys, and navigate the house (as blind dogs quickly learn how to do). Using an olfactory sense that is a million more times acute than a human's,[3] they learn about other dogs' states of being by sniffing where they urinated, and then add their own scent to the mix creating a type of newspaper for the next dog that comes along. They can smell when a door in the house has opened, alerting to the new scents from outdoors, to arrive in time to go for a run, and they can smell out sources of food from great distances. They have even been trained to detect fingerprints on glass six weeks after the glass was touched.[2]

Dogs are so adept at using their sense of smell, that they have been trained as sensors to detect bladder cancer in humans by smelling urine samples, detecting the cancer before any current noninvasive laboratory test is able.[4] They can find microscopic traces of drugs left behind on money, and recently have been trained to find single bed bugs in a building. They are commonly used in searches for missing people and in combat to sniff out explosives and insurgents. Their sense of hearing takes a back seat to the value of the sense of smell in their lives.

Keeping this in mind, owners should not project their own despair at their dog's hearing loss and remind themselves that their dog has other ways to compensate. It is the communication with the owner that suffers most, and that is where owners should concentrate their efforts. For most dogs, a hearing loss can be taken somewhat in stride. On the other hand, for some highly trained dogs who are accustomed to a variety of vocal commands, a hearing loss can be frustrating or cause them to retire early from a career they enjoy.

HEARING LOSS IN CANINES: ARE THERE IMPACT PARALLELS WITH HUMANS?

Before looking at the types of hearing loss, one must question if canine hearing loss has social and emotional parallels to those of humans. Significant permanent hearing loss in humans has a direct impact on academic achievement, vocational success, earned income, social interactions, and family dynamics.[5,6] Studies have further shown that untreated adult human hearing loss is associated with overall poorer health, decreased physical activity, psychosocial dysfunction, and depression.[7,8]

Given the substantial negative impact that hearing loss has within our species, it is understandable that many dog owners become quite concerned when their beloved pet shows signs of diminished hearing. But a legitimate question might be: Does a dog's loss of hearing have the same deleterious effects on quality of life as it does for humans?

As a follow-up, one might further question: Can a dog give and receive the same affections without a sense of hearing? Can a dog harmoniously coexist with its human companions in the presence of hearing loss (in either species)? Can a dog interact joyously with members of its own species when hearing is diminished? The answer to all of these is a reassuring "yes." The greater question is how do we maximize the experience of living with a hearing-impaired or deaf dog? A large answer to this question lies in ensuring adequate communication and safety.

TYPES OF HEARING LOSS

The types of hearing loss in canines parallel the types of hearing loss seen in most other mammals including humans. As discussed elsewhere in this issue, a variety of etiologies can underlie hearing loss, and depending on the pathology, the loss may be amenable to medical intervention. Although the purpose of this article is to provide discussion of management of permanent hearing loss in canines, let us first briefly summarize the types of hearing loss.

Conductive Hearing Loss

Disorders that disrupt the normal sound propagation (or *conduction*) of sound energy from the environment to the cochlea of the inner ear present a conductive hearing loss. Some of these disorders, such as cerumen accumulation in the outer ear canal, otitis externa, and otitis media, are clearly amenable to medical intervention. The sequela of longer-standing, untreated middle ear effusion can result in more permanent hearing deficits. Conductive hearing loss can also arise from disruption or fracture of the middle ear ossicles (the bones that transmit sound vibration from the tympanic membrane to the cochlea) or reduction of ossicle vibration (the stapes in particular) caused by otosclerosis. These latter conditions, although correctable, are difficult to diagnose accurately in canines and are rarely addressed medically. The management discussions in this article, however, can apply to any nonremediated conductive hearing loss.

Sensory Hearing Loss

More permanent hearing loss that affects the cochlear structures (primarily the inner and outer hair cells) can be congenital (present at birth or with delayed onset) or can be adventitious secondary to ototoxic agents, noise exposure, or presbycusis (aging process). Although both sensory and conductive hearing loss create an attenuation of incoming sound intensities, sensory hearing loss creates greater hearing difficulty owing to cochlear distortions even when hearing loss levels (degree of attenuation) are held constant. The effects of sensory hearing loss listed in **Box 1** greatly exacerbate communication difficulties in humans. Given that successful canine

---

Box 1
Effects of sensory hearing loss in humans

Reduced intensity of speech and environmental sounds

Reduced frequency resolution of speech sounds

Reduced temporal resolution of speech sounds

Reduced tolerance for intense sounds

auditory comprehension of human speech is reliant on the accurate reception of a more limited number of brief commands that can partially be deciphered by context and vocal tone, the adverse effects of sensory hearing loss affect canines less.

Mixed Hearing Loss

Mixed hearing loss typically refers to the coexistence of conductive hearing loss and sensory hearing loss. Management is most effective when any treatable conductive component is addressed medically in combination with hearing loss management suggestions presented in this article.

Neural Hearing Loss

Hearing loss that arises from lesions along the cochlear nerve between the cochlea and the brainstem (eg, acoustic neuroma, acoustic neuritis, multiple sclerosis) can produce a neural hearing loss. These hearing losses used to be lumped within the larger term "sensorineural hearing loss"; however, today's diagnostic tools, including measures of auditory brainstem response, recordings of otoacoustic emissions, and imaging through computed tomography scan and magnetic resonance imaging, can differentiate sensory and neural hearing losses, permitting separate classification in humans. In animal audiology, the management of sensory and neural hearing loss is essentially the same, and the 2 types of losses are still routinely classified within the more generic term of sensorineural. Although neural hearing losses are frequently specified as "retrocochlear," it should be noted that by definition this term includes any hearing loss beyond the cochlea; yet, a central hearing loss, which is also beyond the cochlea, is a categorical hearing loss in its own right.

Central (or Cortical) Hearing Loss

A decrease in auditory comprehension in the absence of a concomitant loss of hearing sensitivity is known as a central auditory disorder or auditory processing disorder. The resultant listening difficulties that arise in humans (often resulting in a variety of learning disabilities in schoolchildren) are still frequently undiagnosed or misdiagnosed. Given the vast similarities among animal species' auditory systems, it is likely that some dogs suffer with a central hearing loss; however, the clinical documentation of this disorder within canines would be difficult at best. Although not identified as a disorder, owners of dogs who may have an auditory processing deficit likely recognize that their dogs are easily distracted and side-lined and find means to compensate in their instruction and interactions.

WHAT MIGHT WE EXPECT WITH CANINE HEARING LOSS?

The dog with a congenital hearing loss grows up visually alert and is not truly aware that he is different from other dogs. As discussed earlier, dogs rely on their sense of smell more heavily than their sense of hearing; and for dogs who have hearing loss from birth, there is little we need to do other than to find a mutually satisfactory means to communicate with the animal and ensure its safety and the safety of others.

Dogs who lose their hearing later in life, whether from presbycusis, disease, ototoxic agents, long-term noise exposure, or sudden-impact acoustic trauma, may indeed know that they are different from their compatriots and may sense the loss of hearing more acutely than dogs with congenital hearing loss. It is mostly for these dogs that owners will seek advice from their veterinarian.

The most common questions that the veterinarian may hear from their patient's owners pertain to the warning signs of hearing loss (ie, *What should we be watching for? How do we know there is a loss?*), if the hearing can be tested, and what should be done if a hearing loss is verified.

WHAT ARE THE WARNING SIGNS OF CANINE HEARING LOSS?

In the absence of brain stem auditory evoked response screening (BAER), it is nearly impossible to identify a deaf puppy until after it is weaned. A normally hearing pup will generally begin responding to environmental sounds and voices by about 10 days of age; however, a deaf puppy within a litter of pups lives its early life within the "pack" and will blend with the movements and "group responses" of its littermates. Although a congenitally deaf pup may appear behaviorally more aggressive with its littermates, it is generally only on later separation from the litter that behavioral observations raise suspicion of deafness.

A dog born with a unilateral deafness, or who later acquires a unilateral hearing loss, is more difficult to identify; however, close observation will reveal difficulty localizing the source of sounds and what may appear as a greater disorientation than other dogs. Suspicion of unilateral deafness can only be fully confirmed through BAER testing.

As with humans, as dogs age, their hearing diminishes. This most often is of a gradual onset discovered by owners through observation of changes in the dog's awareness of or responses to environmental sounds or verbal commands.

COMMON SCENARIOS LEADING TO SUSPICION OF ADULT-ONSET BILATERAL HEARING LOSS

Alice arrives home to find her 8-year-old golden retriever, Dixie, happily sleeping on the couch. This would be fine if the dog did not shed all over the couch, she thinks. But her larger concern is that Dixie is usually jumping up and down at the door in happy anticipation before she has even pulled fully into the driveway. As Alice approaches her dreaming dog, her winter boots clomping on the floor, Dixie does not even crack an eye. She reaches down curiously to pet the dog thinking, "Why wasn't she at the door?" As Alice's fingers barely touch fur, Dixie gives a startled yelp and almost bounces off the ceiling. The dog then looks at her with confusion and a sheepish reaction. Dixie does not understand how or why her owner snuck up on her.

Bill is throwing a ball for his border collie, who loses interest for a moment and heads off to sniff a distant tree. Although usually responsive, this time the dog ignores Bill's recall. Finally, in frustration, Bill marches over to the collie and disciplines her for not coming when called. The dog cowers and does not understand what she did wrong or why the playful owner is now angry. She would have come right away if the owner had called!

Max, an 11-year-old show dog and agility champion is in a training session. He knows more than 50 behaviors well, many of them on verbal command. His trainer has noticed that over the past few months some behaviors have become sloppy, or seem to have false starts. In working to tone up these vocally cued behaviors, the dog appears anxious and not as responsive as usual. In later weeks, the dog finally walks away when the trainer gives a series of vocal commands. The dog is willing to work, happy to be trained, and responds well to hand cues, but seems less interested in responding to vocal commands.

These scenarios are often first glimpses into changes in a dog's hearing. Dogs cannot come up to their owners and report that their hearing seems to be failing. It is up to owners to be aware of the changes in their pet's behavior.

For many health problems, changes in behavior can be the first sign. A loss of hearing is no exception. If a dog starts to consistently have a different response than what has been established for years, the owner should consider what may be medically wrong rather than assuming that the dog is misbehaving or lazy.

Most frequently, when questions arise about hearing abilities at a veterinary clinic visit, it is inquiries about an adult dog with adventitious hearing loss, generally from presbycusis. In the absence of any history of otologic disease or excessive noise exposure, such hearing losses are almost always bilateral in nature. Because of the gradual onset of presbycusis, recognizing the signs of bilateral hearing loss in the adult dog is much more difficult than recognizing the signs of bilateral deafness in a puppy. Although the pet owner may have felt that something was not right with their dog for some time, it is most often only after the loss has progressed to significant levels that hearing loss is suspected.

Warning signs of bilateral hearing loss may include the following:

- Sleeping through sounds or a lack of response to sounds for which one would expect a response, such as verbal commands, hand clapping, doorbells, knocks, can opener, car in the driveway (many times breeders suspect a puppy who continues to sleep when the rest of the litter wakes up and runs to greet a person)
- Startling at a touch
- Not responding when called
- Confusion when given previously trained vocal commands
- Startling at loud sounds that in the past were not an issue (eg, owner sneezing, blasts from the TV, a dropped pot) (Note: Some sensory hearing losses decrease sensitivity for soft or average intensity sounds while increasing sensitivity to loud sounds.)
- General decrease in activity level, sleeping more hours in the day than typical for a dog of similar breed and age
- Difficulty waking the dog when sleeping
- Tendency to startle or snap when woken or touched from outside of its field of vision
- Excessive barking or unusual vocal sounds compared with other dogs of comparable age and breed
- Disorientation, confusion, or agitation in familiar settings

Before the onset of universal hearing screening for newborn humans, suspicion of hearing loss was often delayed owing to apparent responses to auditory signals that were actually responses to visual cues accompanying the auditory signal or response to vibrations. These same confounding factors can affect clear identification of hearing loss in the adult dog with true confirmation only possible through BAER testing.

What Should be Done if Hearing Loss is Verified?

As when other maladies arise with one's pets, when canine hearing loss has been confirmed, pet owners/handlers want to know what they can do to improve or restore the dog's quality of life. As stated at the outset of this article, there is frequently considerable projection on the part of owners relative to what hearing loss must mean to their pet. It is likely that the hearing loss is far more disconcerting to the pet owner than it is to the dog; however, there is information that the veterinarian can share that may be beneficial to both the owner and the dog.

Once the owner has pursued any medically appropriate treatment, it is time to find ways to adapt the human/animal relationship to the hearing loss. Teaching the dog to look for eye contact with the owner, and then to pursue hand signals can offer a new and often fun pursuit for the human/dog team, while building communication skills. The owner should be made aware of dangers that accompany a hearing deficit, such as inability to hear cars and other hazards, nonresponsiveness to human speech, nonresponsiveness to expressions of pain and surprise for which a hearing dog may alter behavior, and changes in training to ensure the deafness is taken into consideration, especially involving disciplinary actions.

Considerations When Living with a Hearing-Impaired or Deaf Dog

Life with a hearing-impaired or deaf dog can be quite fulfilling for both the dog and owner; however, there are potential behaviors of which owners should be made aware. Although some of these can be viewed as humorous, others are more directly related to the safety of both family members and the pet.

NOT SO UNIQUE SCENARIOS FROM LIFE WITH A DEAF DOG

Linda, who had owned her congenitally deaf Australian Shepherd named Belle for about 6 months, relays a story of mistaken identity. Linda was in the shower with the window open on a beautiful summer morning when she heard a woman calling from the deck outside the kitchen. Sticking her head out of the curtain, she listened again, "Yoo Who!" Linda called out, "Crissy, is that you?" But there was no response. A moment later she heard a repeat call, "Yoooo Whooooo!" This time Linda called "Crissy, come on in! I'll be out in a minute!" Still, no response. "Yoooooooo Whoooooooo?" Feeling slightly perplexed that she could not make herself heard, Linda got out of the shower, dripping wet, wrapped herself in a large towel and went to the door to greet her friend. To her surprise her friend was not there. Instead she saw Belle through the kitchen window happily calling "Yoooooo Whoooo!" Living with a deaf dog has many challenges...some are indeed comical, as in this scenario, which shows how unusual some of the sounds are that a congenitally deaf dog can make.

Sometimes those unusual sounds can cause owners embarrassment. Ted and Alice took their deaf golden retriever to their children's cross-country meet. Dixie was one of many dogs in attendance. They lined up with dozens of other parents and spectators along a lightly wooded path where all the runners would pass. As the first runners came through, Dixie became excited. By the time their own kids came through, she wanted to run along and showed her displeasure of the leash by SCREAMING. This was not a dog whine or howl, but rather nonstop blood-curdling, drawn out soprano SCREAMS right out of an old movie with the heroine tied on the railroad tracks. All eyes turned toward Ted and Alice with silent accusations of torture. There was just no way to explain what was going on to that many people, so they slunk away as quickly as they could.

Unfortunately, a deaf dog cannot hear our unexpected sounds. A dog with normal hearing takes notice when its human is displeased. For example, Rhonda was lying in bed reading a book when her 95-pound deaf shepherd, Mackenzie, jumped onto the bed, landing on the owners' stomach. Although a dog with normal hearing gets the picture not to do that again without much actual training, a deaf dog will never hear its owner's "OOF" and grunt and will remain completely oblivious to the discomfort caused by jumping up on the bed. Although Rhonda's dog may not learn from this, Rhonda surely will learn to expect another unexpected gut punch.

A deaf dog will not hear a person yelp if play gets too rough. If the dog has not been taught properly, and rough play is encouraged, a deaf dog may assume it can play as roughly with a human as with another dog. Human skin is not as pliable or resilient as canine skin, and injuries can happen. When playing with a child, the dog will not hear the discomfort of the child and may think the child's attempts to fend it off are just more play, increasing the risk. Even more than with a hearing dog, care must be taken from the start to teach good manners to a deaf dog.

Dogs pay attention to the sounds and behaviors of other dogs to determine attitude and whether an encounter will be friendly or aggressive. A growl is an aggressive sound, a whine is a plea, a yip is an invitation to play, and so forth. If a deaf dog gets into a fight with another dog, it will not hear when the other dog yelps, whines, or makes submissive "you win" sounds. Because submission is also usually shown by exposure of the throat and belly, a dog submitting in the fight is at risk if the deaf dog does not accept the submission, as it was not heard. Deaf dogs are not any more violent than hearing dogs, but a deaf dog is still biologically/instinctually wired, exactly the same as a hearing dog, to expect certain behaviors. The deaf dog lacks the self-awareness to realize it will never receive the full submission (sound and exposure).

Ryan's story exemplifies the inherent dangers of when a deaf dog fails to recognize submission. Ryan's border collie, "Q," was very hard on the family's deaf dog, Beethoven. Q felt she had to be in charge all the time, bullying Beethoven. Ryan and his wife, Lucy, intervened and maintained the peace for years, but one Sunday night Q snapped at Beethoven, slightly scratching Beethoven's nose. Beethoven responded with a full charge. Q immediately realized she was in trouble, whimpered and rolled onto her back, but Beethoven was on her, clamping down on multiple places and shaking for all he was worth. Q was crying out and submitting, but Beethoven was not responding and continued to bite and shake violently. The owners separated them as quickly as possible...the fight lasted just moments...but poor Q spent the night in the hospital, was very sore for days, and Ryan and Lucy were out more than $1000 in veterinary bills.

Last year, Ryan and Lucy added a rescued 9-month-old beagle to their home. Beethoven had a difficult time comprehending the new hound's behaviors. The beagle, "Bones," would run up to Beethoven and bay. At first Beethoven thought the running at him, raising the head so high, and opening the mouth at him were signs of aggression from Bones. But as soon as Beethoven would start to react, Bones would go into a play bow, roll over or run off, completely confusing the deaf dog. It took a few months, but Bones taught Beethoven to play like a dog, which was a joy Beethoven could never share with Q.

Dog Owner/Handler Communication with the Hearing-Impaired or Deaf Dog

Deaf dogs learn quickly to watch faces and learn to associate their owner's moods with the corresponding facial expressions. Savvy owners can use this to their advantage. Because the dog understands the angry face, sometimes that is all that is needed to get a point across. Owners have to take care to send consistent messages. It can be hard to keep an angry face while scolding, when one just wants to laugh at all the feathers stuck onto the furry face that got into the school art project. But if the owner laughs and smiles, the deaf dog may pick up on that more than the scolding, and dive right back into the feathers for more fun.

Dogs have been bred by humans for tens of thousands of years for many specific traits: herding, guarding, body size, nose length, color, ear size, temperament, coat type, webbed feet, tail shape, amount of wrinkles in the skin.....the list goes on and on. One trait that is true across the board, regardless of breed, is that we want our dogs to be in tune with people. We want them to accept humans as their pack and to look to us for guidance. This quality is what makes the domestic dog such a good pet, and a wonderful companion and working partner. This is also the quality that allows us to create an interspecies communication system.

Deaf dogs are just as intelligent and willing as hearing dogs. Dogs are hardwired to communicate. They instinctually use facial expressions and body language, in addition to sounds. These expressions would be of no use to a dog if no other dog could "read" them. Dogs are able, willing, and actually very perceptive at reading human facial expressions and body language. They also have their hidden ace; that sense of smell that helps to cue them in on how we are feeling.

Dogs that are congenitally deaf learn quickly to watch for facial signs in the people around them to help them understand situations. This is a natural survival instinct. A deaf dog that is socialized properly with humans will watch faces and body language and learn to change its behavior based on what it reads in the people. Dogs that become deaf later in life already know the basics and have had the advantage of formerly heard sounds that have taught them what frame of mind may be paired with which human facial expression and body language. With their hearing not helping them, they naturally look for additional information by watching more.

This natural ability to read humans gives us a wonderful basis for communication. Deaf dogs can be taught a wide range of visual cues. These cues can be hand signs (a form of dog sign language), owner body position, blinking lights, prop driven commands, and so forth. Many owners train their dogs to visual cues without even realizing it, such as when the owner puts on a coat and the dog begins dancing around the owner asking for a walk.

As with all training, consistency is the key. With deaf dogs, this includes consistency of body language and facial expression. As in the example with the feathers, training will be slowed or confused by mixed signals. Explicit training can commence once the deaf dog has an established, healthy relationship with the owner.

Owners can use food reward, toy reward, affection, or combinations to keep the dog interested in the training. Training should be performed in a positive atmosphere, with the goal being enjoyable, useful communication. A good start is to train a recall. Have the dog loose in an enclosed area. Have some treats available. When the dog looks up, show it a treat and make the gesture you want to use that means "come here." Any visual cue should be easy to remember, easy to perform, and easily distinguished from other cues. In the case of "come," a visual cue easily understood from a long distance is advisable. When the dog comes over for the treat, the owner should be aware to show a happy facial expression, make eye contact with the dog, and praise it with affection while giving the treat. Soon the dog will be watching for the visual hand cue, and excited to come when it sees it. This can easily be paired with a light cue, such as a flashlight turning on and off, or blinking outside lights, so that a deaf dog loose in a yard can be recalled at night even when not directly looking at the owner.

This same method is used to train a deaf dog to come to the vibration of a collar. The owner shows the dog a treat and as the dog comes to get it, the owner vibrates the collar. Once the dog is not surprised by the collar vibration, and the treat has made the vibration a positive experience, the owner vibrates the collar simultaneously with showing the treat. The dog learns to associate the vibration with the food reward. Eventually, the vibration alone will alert the dog to return to the owner for a reward.

The basic principle is the same for each trained visual cue. Pair visual cues with behaviors and communication, and reward when the dog responds appropriately. Dogs quickly pick up signs for suppertime, time to go outside (bathroom break), back up, sit down, stay, look at me, look over there, put that down, give that to me, do you want to play? They can even be taught signs for individual toys. Just as importantly, dogs learn the sign for NO! This sign should be very clear, very distinct, easily and quickly made with one hand, and accompanied with an angry face. We use the classic, side to side, scolding index finger.

Disciplining deaf dogs can be more challenging than disciplining hearing dogs. For example, Dan is relaxing in the living room when he looks up and sees his young deaf dog, Suzie, stealing some meat off the kitchen counter. He yells and runs to the kitchen. A hearing dog would have heard the angry yell as it took the meat. In this case, Suzie has swallowed the free meat that her owner obviously was not guarding for himself, never heard the yelling, was very happy with her treat, and is now beginning to scratch an itch. All of a sudden she is being hit, and Dan is there with a very angry expression. She is surprised and scared and reacts by trying to twist away. She cannot get away, she hurts from where she was hit, her owner looks and smells scary. She is confused, and finally attempts a bite in her panic. This further infuriates Dan and the situation continues to go downhill. Suzie never does understand what went wrong…she was just scratching herself! Damage has been done to the relationship, and if Dan does not learn how to communicate better, Suzie is going to start biting to protect herself.

Owners of deaf dogs need to be proactive, especially while their dogs are young and learning the rules of living with humans. The best solution to Suzie's dilemma would be for the meat to not be accessible in the first place. Leaving it out invites Suzie to learn that the counter is a good place to find treats. Let's look at a different way for Dan to deal with Suzie.

Dan looks up in time to see Suzie stealing the meat off the counter. Understanding that he will not get there in time, and that this is a training situation, Dan keeps his temper under control but quickly makes it over to Suzie. He lays another piece of meat at the edge of the counter, stands back and waits. Suzie smells the meat, reaches for it, but is immediately intercepted by Dan, who puts on a very angry expression and gives her a strong visual cue for NO! If necessary, he can hold her muzzle gently but firmly while making her watch the NO cue. Then Dan makes her leave the room, removes any easily stolen food, and monitors Suzie for a while to make her stay near him in the living room, effectively giving her a time out by limiting her freedom. Suzie realizes she got in trouble while reaching for the meat, knows her owner is mad and why, and realizes that she has lost some freedom while her owner is angry. They have communicated, no damage was done to the relationship, and Suzie has taken a step in learning the rules.

There are other "tricks" that can be used as long-distance disciplines, or to get a deaf dog's attention. Some owners believe a squirt gun is best for getting attention. An Airzooka can also be used with good success. This drum-sized toy shoots a powerful slug of air about 30 ft, enough to startle a dog a room away and cause the dog to look over to the owner, who can redirect the dog away from the mischief.

KEEPING THE HEARING-IMPAIRED OR DEAF DOG SAFE

A deaf dog cannot hear a car racing down the street, and cannot hear a warning or recall issued by the owner. It is difficult to keep a loose deaf dog safe. An owner who wishes to take a deaf dog off leash may have success communicating a recall with a vibration collar. Vibration collars are available through distributors for hunting dog training aids. The collar can be set to vibrate when the owner pushes a button, alerting the dog that the owner is recalling. Care has to be taken that the dog does not get out of range where the collar will no longer respond to the handset. The owner must spend many hours training the deaf dog to respond to the collar consistently.

Because it is more difficult to get a deaf dog back if it gets loose, other precautions can increase the chances of keeping the dog safe. Always have owner information attached to the dog's collar so that if someone finds the deaf dog, the dog can be brought home. Micro-chipping is another good safety measure. Even if the dog loses its collar, a microchip can still bring it home.

Physical fencing is always a great option for keeping pets home and safely confined. In some subdivisions, physical fencing is prohibited and invisible fencing (electronic fencing, usually involving a shock collar) may offer a solution, but only when used in appropriate circumstances. Although the use of such "fencing" may be a convenience for dog owners, there are added risks over conventional fencing. Without appropriate supervision of the dog at all times, in conjunction with knowledgeable, proper training to the fence to keep shocking at an absolute minimum, dogs will sometimes run through the fence or be traumatized by the training. Furthermore, hearing dogs are able to listen for an audible beep, warning the dog that they are approaching the perimeter. When choosing an invisible fence company, owners of deaf dogs must be assured that the collar has a vibration setting to warn the dog of the perimeter and must train accordingly. If the owner is already using a vibration collar as a recall device, this can cause confusion. Unlike physical barriers, invisible fences keep your pet in, but do not keep other dogs out. Owners must be diligent not to leave a pet "safely" in the yard, just to have it attacked by a loose dog.

Audiological Management of the Hearing-Impaired or Deaf Dog

In human audiology, audiologists are not only interested in determining the extent and impact of an existing hearing loss, an equally important test outcome is differentiating the site of lesion of the hearing difficulty (conductive, sensory, neural, or central). In canines, the primary evaluation concern is ascertaining the degree of hearing loss and the amount of residual hearing abilities.

If hearing aid amplification is being considered for a dog, we require specific testing to determine audiological "candidacy" of a dog. As with human amplification, dogs require a certain amount of residual hearing for amplification to be effective. To be considered for amplification, we require candidates to have BAER with insert earphone delivery no poorer than 102 dB peSPL (equivalent to 80 dB nHL) using an IHS testing unit (Intelligent Hearing Systems, Miami, FL). The waveforms must contain at least waves I, II, III, and V and must be replicated using 2000 sweeps at either 17.1 or 33.3 clicks per second using a condensation or alternating stimulus with filter settings of 100 Hz and 1500 Hz. If the candidate has a hearing loss no worse than our cutoff criteria, then the same test is run in a free-field (through speakers) in an audiological sound booth to attain unaided BAER responses that can be later compared with aided BAER responses.

Based on the set criteria, and if the dog and owners are good candidates with respect to commitment and behavior, silicone impressions of the ears are taken for laboratory fabrication into hearing aids. Once the hearing aids are received from the hearing aid laboratory, the dog is fitted with them and the free-field BAER testing is run again with hearing aids. This final testing process allows for "tuning" of the hearing aids to ensure improved audibility.

At the University of Cincinnati's FETCH~LAB (www.fetchlab.org), we have been experimenting with canine amplification for the past several years with very mixed results. Otter, the first dog we fit with hearing aids, was our most successful. Not coincidentally, Otter was probably the most highly trained dog we have worked with. He had appeared on David Letterman's Stupid Pet Tricks and several TV shows, performed regularly, and knew more than 100 behaviors.

BAER testing revealed Otter had a severe hearing loss bilaterally (approximately 70 dB nHL). Otter's hearing loss was secondary to presbycusis and his animal trainer/ owners sensed that he appeared stressed that he could no longer discern verbal commands. He was outfitted with digital postauricular human hearing aids attached to a cowl (**Fig. 1**). Fairly lengthy tubing extended from the hearing aids to custom-fabricated Lucite earmolds fitted to each ear.

As expected, Otter did not at first recognize hearing aid–amplified sound as something meaningful. It took considerable consistent behavioral conditioning for Otter to wear the hearing aids for increasing lengths of time. Eventually he became aware that he was missing something when the hearing aids were not worn and he began to re-recognize the verbal commands he had responded to when his hearing was normal.

The "ah HA!" moment for Otter came during a training session after weeks of wearing the aids. After performing several behaviors for hand cues, his trainer set him up for what used to be a favorite behavior in which Otter had to wait for a verbal command from a prone position. He had become increasingly frustrated with this behavior over the past few years as he lost his hearing. This time he heard the verbal command and was so surprised that at the first command, he jumped to his feet and spun toward the trainer. Setting the behavior up a second time, Otter exploded into the behavior, then ran excitedly to the trainer and happily repeated the behavior over and

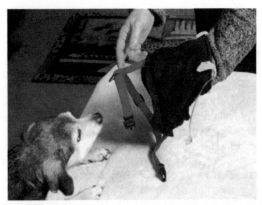

Fig. 1. Following protracted and dedicated training, this highly skilled dog adapted to use of amplification and sought his hearing aids in the morning. Hearing aids provided by ReSound (Bloomington, MN). (Custom earmolds *courtesy of* Westone Laboratories, Colorado Springs, CO.) (*Courtesy of* University of Cincinnati FETCH~LAB, Cincinnati, OH.)

over. After that, he accepted the hearing aids easily and would wear them 10 hours or more each day, napping and running outside without removing them. He would even come looking for his cowl in the morning, tugging it off a table and standing stock still so that the hearing aids could be put on.

As stated, Otter was our most successful fitting. Yet even with his success, questions remain. Otter, unfortunately died of cancer, within 6 months after he received his hearing aids. It is unknown if he would have continued to wear his hearing aids or if he would have instead begun to rely more on visual cues and signs for communication with his owner/trainer. Dogs are very resilient, do not communicate primarily through audition, and most frequently do continue with their lives quite successfully in the presence of diminished hearing.

Subsequent hearing aid fittings were done with custom-molded completely in the concha hearing aids equipped with wireless microphone transmission to convey the owner's voice directly to the dog's ear at distances up to 50 ft (**Fig. 2**). In spite of the higher level of technology, the dogs fit with this device were not as successful as Otter, most likely as postfitting training was not as diligent.

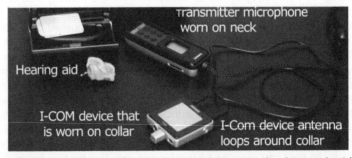

Fig. 2. Custom Phonak (Warrenville, IL) hearing aid (worn in the dog's ear) with wireless transmitter microphone (worn by dog owner) and I-COM receiver (worn on the dog's collar). Owner's voice can be transmitted up to 30 ft. (*Courtesy of* University of Cincinnati FETCH~LAB, Cincinnati, OH.)

What have we learned from our experiences? With hearing aid fittings on subsequent dogs, we have discovered the following:

- When canine hearing loss develops, it is the owner, not the dog, who is being "treated" when we fit hearing aids.
- The owner must either be a skilled trainer or work closely under the guidance of an animal behaviorist if the hearing aids are to be tolerated.
- A behaviorist can give owners training steps to take *before* hearing aids are pursued, both to assess the ability of the owner/dog team to successfully complete the training, and to pretrain the dog to accept a device.
- Training, as in all other areas, must be consistent and is expected to be long term.
- The dog must have a history of being easily trained and compliant.
- The owner must have the patience of Job.

Even with these factors all in place, success is a relative term in canine amplification and never guaranteed. We have learned that the first approach when owners want hearing aids for their dogs (and FETCH ~ LAB gets calls weekly) is serious counseling with the owners so that they know who they are getting hearing aids for (it is really more for the owner than for the dog), what will be expected from the owner, and that life with a hearing-impaired dog can be highly enjoyable and rewarding in spite of the hearing loss without hearing aids.

Other Amplification Options

Dog owners frequently inquire if implanted amplification may be more successful with dogs. The underlying thought is, given that much of the requisite training with the dog is geared toward acceptance of having something foreign in the ear canal, an implanted device may be more successful. There are caveats for each of the 3 implanted approaches.

- Osseointegrated Auditory Implant (aka: Bone-Anchored Hearing Aids): Bone-anchored hearing aids are used for conductive hearing losses or mixed hearing losses with a large conductive component. As such, they are not truly applicable for dogs with gradual-onset, presbycusic hearing loss, as the requisite bone conduction (neural reserve) is lacking. From an audiologic perspective alone, this style hearing aid could be considered for dogs with conductive hearing loss secondary to ear disease. However, other factors would still rule this out for canine implantation.

  The actual processor is attached to a surgically implanted titanium post in the mastoid bone. The cost of bone-anchored hearing aids for humans is approximately $3000 for the titanium implant itself. When one adds to this the cost of surgery and the surgical and audiological aftercare, cost alone is not a small consideration when considering this device for canines. The sound processors of these devices are more sensitive to damage from extreme weather conditions than are more traditional hearing devices. Of a greater concern are the reported incidents when a blow to the head during sports has broken the anchor from the bone in humans. This certainly makes the device inappropriate for canines.
- Middle-Ear Implants: Middle-ear implants have some advantages over traditional hearing aids but come at a considerable cost: as high as $15,000 for the device and surgical procedure. Side effects reported in humans with middle-ear implants have included partial facial paralysis and loss of taste.
- Cochlear Implantation: A cochlear implant provides stimulation directly to the cochlear nerve, bypassing the damaged hair cells in the cochlea that no longer stimulate the cochlear nerve. The average cost for a cochlear implant for human

deafness, including preimplant evaluations, the implant itself, surgery, and post-operative aural rehabilitation, is more than $40,000. Without being able to fine-tune the device with clear input from the canine, it is questionable how successful a cochlear implant might be.

HEARING LOSS PREVENTION

Up to this point, this article has been addressing existing hearing loss and its management. The prevention of avoidable hearing loss should be of equal importance to veterinarians and dog owners/handlers. Although hearing loss is inevitable with the aging process, hearing loss for younger canines is often preventable.

The adverse effects of noise exposure on human hearing are well documented and have culminated in legislation for the protection of workers' hearing. The Occupational Safety and Health Administration[9] and the National Institute of Occupational Health[10] have both set guidelines for hearing protection from noise exposure that permits a time-intensity trade-off in which a worker's permissible exposure level decreases as the length of exposure time increases.

Canines, too, can be at risk of hearing damage from excess sound levels, but their hearing is not protected through damage-risk legislation. Although FETCH~LAB research has documented that the intensity of driers commonly used during dog grooming is sufficiently loud to damage the groomer's hearing, the shorter duration of exposure for the dog being groomed renders the intensity safe for canines. In contrast, given the longer exposure times, FETCH~LAB has demonstrated that the noise levels in kennels can damage the hearing of dogs kenneled for longer periods of time.[11] Working dogs in the military are frequently exposed to noise levels for which their handlers are afforded hearing protection. The FETCH~LAB is currently working toward proposed solutions to help protect the hearing of these highly trained animals.

"Civilian" dogs are not routinely exposed to intense noise. All advocates for canine health and safety, however, should promote awareness of potential dangers to canine hearing. The FETCH~LAB successfully installed sound-absorbing panels in a local kennel to mitigate noise levels. Hunters who wear hearing protection should be cognizant of the proximity of their dogs to gunfire and consider protecting their dog's hearing as they should their own. Effective canine hearing protection is currently under development through the University of Cincinnati FETCH~LAB.

SUMMARY

Dog owners and handlers are naturally concerned when suspicion of hearing loss arises for their dogs. Questions frequently asked of the veterinarian center on warning signs of canine hearing loss and what can be done for the dog if hearing loss is confirmed. Communication training and safety awareness issues should be paramount for those living with a hearing-impaired or deaf dog. Some owners/handlers will ask about the feasibility of hearing aid use for their dog. Given the many obstacles to success in this arena, hearing aid use is generally not recommended. Although hearing loss is inevitable for dogs as they age, as it is for humans, owners should be aware of potential damaging noises their animals may be exposed to and possible means to prevent noise-induced hearing loss in canines.

REFERENCES

1. Watson L. Jacobson's organ and the remarkable nature of smell. New York: Penguin Putnam Inc; 2001.

2. Houpt KA. Domestic animal behavior for veterinarians & animal scientists. 5th edition. Ames (IA): Wiley-Blackwell; 2011.
3. Campbell KL, Corbin JE, Campbell JR. Companion animals, their biology, care, health and management. New Jersey: Pearson Prentice Hall; 2005.
4. Olfactory detection of human bladder cancer by dogs: proof of principle study. BMJ 2004;329. http://dx.doi.org/10.1136/bmj.329.7468.712.
5. Northern JL, Downs MP. Hearing in children. 4th edition. Baltimore (MD): Williams and Wilkins; 1991.
6. National American Precis Syndicated. (2007). Money matters: hearing loss may mean income loss. Available at: www.napsnet.com/health/70980.html. Accessed July 10, 2007.
7. Bess F, Lichtenstein J, Logan S, et al. Hearing impairment as a detriment of function in the elderly. J Am Geriatr Soc 1989;37:123–8.
8. Chisolm TH, Johnson CE, Danhauer JL, et al. American Academy of Audiology task force of the health-related quality of life benefits of amplification in adults. J Am Acad Audiol 2007;18:151–83.
9. Occupational Safety, Health Administration. Occupational noise exposure: hearing conservation amendment; final rule. Fed Regist 1983;46:9738–85.
10. Criteria for a recommended standard: occupational noise exposure (report No. 98–126.). Cincinnati (OH): National Institute of Occupational Safety and Health; 1998. Author.
11. Scheifle P, Martin D, Clark JG, et al. Impact of kennel noise on canine hearing. Am J Vet Res 2012;73:482–9.

Electrodiagnostic Evaluation of Auditory Function in the Dog

Peter M. Scheifele, PhD[a,b,c],*, John Greer Clark, PhD[a]

KEYWORDS

- Electrophysiology • Canine hearing loss • Brainstem auditory evoked response
- BAER test • Auditory evoked potential • Otoacoustic emission
- Auditory steady state response

KEY POINTS

- Given the high incidence of deafness within several breeds of dogs, accurate hearing screening and assessment is essential.
- In addition to brainstem auditory evoked response (BAER) testing, 2 other electrophysiologic tests are now being examined as audiologic tools for use in veterinary medicine: otoacoustic emissions and the auditory steady state response (ASSR).
- To improve BAER testing of animals and ensure an accurate interpretation of test findings from one test site to another, the establishment of and adherence to clear protocols is essential.
- The ASSR is not used in screening but rather when a more comprehensive hearing assessment is needed.
- The ASSR holds promise as an objective test for rapid testing of multiple frequencies in both ears simultaneously.
- Otoacoustic emissions (OAEs) are clinically important as rapid, non-invasive tests that can be done in any one of three modalities: frequency, distortion product, and transient function.
- OAEs are directly related to the cochlear amplification function.

INTRODUCTION

Canine hearing assessment is important for screening breeds that are commonly afflicted with congenital deafness. Congenital deafness has been reported in more than 90 breeds.[1] Demonstrating normal hearing thresholds is also critical for working and service dogs to determine whether they can respond appropriately to

The authors have nothing to disclose.
[a] Department of Communication Sciences and Disorders, University of Cincinnati, 3202 Eden Avenue, Cincinnati, OH 45106, USA; [b] Department of Neuroaudiology and Neuroanatomy, University of Cincinnati, 3202 Eden Avenue, Cincinnati, OH 45106, USA; [c] Department of Medical Education, University of Cincinnati, 3202 Eden Avenue, Cincinnati, OH 45106, USA
* Corresponding author. 3104 Ninnichuck Road, Bethel, OH 45106.
E-mail address: scheifpr@ucmail.uc.edu

environmental auditory cues. Finally, diagnostic testing of auditory function and acuity is necessary for detecting presbycusis (age-related hearing loss) and ear pathologies, such as primary secretory otitis media (PSOM), and to identify progressive or acquired hearing impairments to long-term noise exposure (eg, kennel noise) or repeated, sudden-intense impact noise exposure.

The auditory brainstem response (ABR) is an electrophysiologic test used in humans and animal species to objectively assess auditory function and estimate hearing acuity. These electrophysiologic measures are a more accurate alternative to observing a Preyer reflex, the moving back of the ears seen in some animals in response to an unexpected suprathreshold noise. In addition, behavioral/observational testing cannot be used for diagnostic purposes or to test for unilateral hearing loss.[1–3]

First described by Jewett and Williston in 1971,[4] the ABR records neural activity generated in the cochlear nerve and brain stem in response to a controlled sound stimulus. In humans, the ABR is used for screening newborn hearing, estimating hearing thresholds, localizing some neurologic lesions, monitoring the integrity of auditory pathways during neurosurgical procedures, and noninvasive experimental study of the human auditory system. ABRs are considered the primary yardstick for determining hearing abnormalities in infants.[2] The ABR, also referred to in the literature relating to animals as the *brainstem auditory evoked response* (BAER), evaluates hearing in each ear independently and can be obtained reliably when the patient is awake, sedated, or anesthetized.[1,5,6] This article refers to this electrophysiologic test as the ABR when referring to testing of humans, and the BAER when referring to animal screening and evaluation.

Two other electrophysiologic tests that are now being examined as audiologic tools for use in veterinary medicine are otoacoustic emissions (OAEs) and the auditory steady state response (ASSR). These tests are commonly used in humans to diagnose cochlear dysfunction and to better estimate hearing acuity.[2,3,5] When used in conjunction with BAER testing, OAEs may be a more accurate method for hearing screening. The ASSR is a new technique that is an objective frequency-specific approach to estimate hearing acuity.

The purpose of this article is to

- Outline BAER instrumentation and recording techniques,
- Discuss the use of BAER testing for hearing screening and diagnostic purposes,
- Provide an overview of OAE testing,
- Discuss the combined use of OAE testing with BAER testing for complete auditory clinical assessment, and
- Provide an overview of the ASSR.

USE OF BAER TESTING IN VETERINARY MEDICINE

In veterinary clinical practice, BAER testing is mainly used as a screening mechanism; however, it also has great potential as a diagnostic tool for central auditory dysfunction.[7,8] In dogs, the BAER test is commonly used to certify that puppies are free from congenital hereditary deafness. The Orthopedic Foundation for Animals recognizes the BAER test as the only acceptable testing modality for diagnosing canine deafness.[9] In addition to screening for congenital hereditary deafness, the BAER test can help estimate canine hearing thresholds and is useful for diagnosing various forms of canine deafness. Serial BAER testing of working and service dogs can be used to identify progressive or acquired hearing impairments subsequent to presbycusis, long-term noise exposure (eg, kennel noise), or repeated, sudden-intense impact noise exposure.

A NEED FOR STANDARDIZED BAER PROTOCOL

Since the 1971 publication by Jewett and Williston[4] on ABR, a large amount of material has been published regarding the clinical and research importance of ABRs in humans and the BAER in various animal species.[1,5,10] Although BAER testing is proving to be valuable in veterinary medicine, its usefulness beyond puppy screening remains questionable for diagnostic purposes. Assessment of BAER in the dog depends on the comparison of an individual dog's BAERs with appropriately matched normative data. These data have been published for air-conducted click stimuli, air-conducted tone-burst stimuli, and bone-conducted click stimuli, but the stimulus and recording parameters are not consistent in any of these previous studies because of the lack of agreement of universally accepted clinical norms. Without these norms, tests performed by one clinician cannot be duplicated by another, and lack a basis for accurate diagnosis based solely on waveform morphology analysis. This issue is well-known by audiologists given that human audiology historically had similar challenges in its infancy.[2,3] Therefore, keeping in line with human audiology, protocol for establishing normative data in the dog for BAER testing would include standardized click presentation rate and bandwidth filter settings, and the use of peak-equivalent sound pressure level reference (peSPL) in place of a normalized hearing level reference (nHL).

AUDITORY EVOKED POTENTIALS: BAER TESTING MECHANICS, INSTRUMENTATION, AND TECHNIQUES

The brain responds to repetitive sensory stimuli through consistent and time-locked changes in electrical activity, which can be recorded from electrodes placed in the scalp. These readings are referred to as *evoked responses*, and the waveform responses recorded early, within the first 10 ms, are referred to as the *BAER*.[11] The BAER is a far-field recording of electrical events, and provides a measure of neural responses from the cranial nerve VIII and lower brainstem auditory nuclei. The response in small animals consists of up to 7 waves, although only the first 5 are clinically relevant (**Fig. 1**). The positive peaks are labeled with Roman numerals. The exact generator sites that are specific to each of the waves observed in a BAER have not been confirmed with certainty.[1,12,13] However, the fifth peak, known as wave V, is

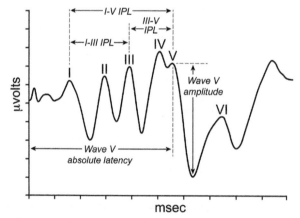

Fig. 1. Example of a normal BAER. Peaks are labeled sequentially with Roman numerals (I–VI). IPL, interpeak latency; msec, milliseconds. (*Courtesy of* Dr L.K. Cole and Mr T. Vojt, The Ohio State University, Columbus, OH.)

usually the most prominent wave, with a large amplitude and negative trough following the positive peak.[14,15] Currently it is accepted that wave I derives from the distal portion of cranial nerve VIII, wave II from the proximal portion of cranial nerve VIII, wave III from the cochlear nuclei, and waves IV and V from multiple generator sites, including the inferior colliculus and perhaps the medial geniculate body; however, in practicality, the latter makes no good electrical sense.

Current BAER equipment is computer-based and can be divided into recording and stimulus components. The recording components consist of recording electrodes, differential amplifier, signal averager, and display screen, whereas the stimulus components include a stimulus generator and a transducer.[16]

Equipment

Recording components

Amplifier Because of the small amplitude of the BAER waveform, which is measured in microvolts, the signal requires considerable amplification. An absolute gain setting of 100,000 to 150,000 is typically used. The amplifier is set to record in the microvolt range.

Filters The purpose of the band-pass filter is to eliminate noise (artifact) without eliminating the BAER response and to improve the signal-to-noise ratio (SNR). High-pass filters pass frequencies higher than their cutoff frequency, whereas low-pass filters pass frequencies lower than their cutoff frequency. The high-pass cutoff should be set at 300 Hz, and the low band-pass filter is set at 1.5 kHz. A filter is either a hardware or software device that provides frequency-dependent transmission or exclusion of energy within bands of interest.

Signal averager The raw signal recorded from the scalp electrodes also typically contains 60 Hz of electrical noise from muscle contraction, the dog's brain activity, and external power sources.[14,17] Because the auditory evoked potentials used to elicit the BAER are much smaller than the electrical noise, this unwanted signal must be isolated from the background electroencephalogram.[6] Each time a click stimulus or tone pip/tone burst (pure tone of the desired audiometric frequency that has a defined start [rise time], duration [plateau], and end [fall time]) is presented and data are recorded, one sweep occurs.[2] The resultant BAER is obtained through averaging a set number of sweeps or repetitions.[3,14] Averaging the responses over multiple stimulus repetitions or sweeps decreases the background noise, making the BAER waves more visible.[3,5] These time-locked auditory evoked potentials remain constant for all stimuli and become amplified across many repetitions, whereas the random background noise detected by the electrodes[3] varies and is reduced through averaging the number of sweeps.[14,17] Therefore, the appropriate number of sweeps is determined based on how many repetitions are needed during signal averaging to produce an adequate SNR for confident visual detection of wave V.[3,17]

Typically, 1000 to 2000 sweeps for each BAER at each stimulus level should be run to ensure that the results accurately represent the function of the central auditory nervous system.[1,3,5] Poor BAER waveforms resulting from high-frequency electrical noise or muscle artifact noise from subject movement can sometimes be improved through increasing the number of sweeps.[3]

Stimulus components

Stimulus type BAERs are generally acquired using a 100-μs broadband click stimulus with 12,000-Hz bandwidth power spectra as tested by sound analysis software. Although this click contains energy in the range of 500 to 4000 Hz, it effectively stimulates the 2000- to 4000-Hz region of the cochlea in humans and animals.

Stimuli for performing BAER testing may also include the use of tone pips/tone bursts. The maximum frequency at which hearing can be tested with most equipment is 14,000 Hz, dictated by the transducer capabilities, unless the equipment has high-frequency extension software and associated transducers. An exception would be the use of special ultrasonic transducers (such as on mice), but this is not done on dogs.

Stimulus polarity Polarity refers to the starting phase of the BAER that affects the direction of the output waveform.[1,3] Stimulus polarity determines the initial waveform morphology, wave amplitudes, and latencies. Most commercial evoked potential instruments allow a choice of condensation, rarefaction, or alternating polarity. Condensation is the polarity that initially causes the pressure wave of the transducer to move toward the eardrum. Rarefaction is the stimulus polarity that causes the initial pressure wave front of the transducer to move away from the tympanic membrane.[3] Condensation stimuli increase polarization of cochlear hair cells, whereas rarefaction activates or depolarizes hair cells within the cochlea, producing BAERs with shorter latencies and larger amplitudes.[3] In humans, rarefaction clicks have been shown to generate a clearer response more frequently than condensation.[3] Alternating polarity alternates between condensation and rarefaction. The stimulus polarity used for testing can result in latency changes for wave V.[3] In human audiology, the recommendation is to use the same polarity for ABR testing as was used to collect the normative data.[2] and the American Society of Clinical Neurophysiology guidelines state that the polarity followed by the user must be indicated in the data results.[18]

Stimulus rate The stimulus presentation rate is a significant stimulus parameter variable[3] that denotes the number of stimuli presented per unit of time.[3,5,9] The overall objective in selecting the stimulus presentation rate when performing the BAER is to present the stimuli as fast as possible without affecting waveform quality or repeatability.[3,5,19] Increasing the stimulus presentation rate has been shown to increase BAER latencies and reduce amplitudes and waveform reproducibility,[3,5,9,14,19] whereas slower repetition rates tend to preserve waveform morphology.[2]

If the click rate is too fast, the auditory pathway reaches an adapted state after a few stimuli and no further changes will be noted despite exposure to additional clicks.[14] The presentation rate of the stimulus must be slow enough to avoid neural adaptation but high enough for efficient data collection.[3,20] Adjusting the stimulus rate can reduce the appearance of electrical artifact in the waveform.[3] As repetition rate is increased, waveform morphology quality is reduced.[2] Even though slower rates provide better morphology, faster repetition rates can be used to expedite threshold testing.[2]

In humans, increasing the stimulus rate up to 30 clicks per second has minimal impact on the ABR waveform.[3,5,9] Infants are routinely screened using rates up to 39.1 clicks per second,[2] whereas a rate of 20 clicks per second is used in adults.[3] An odd number of stimulus rates is advisable to reduce interference with the 60-Hz electrical noise.[2,3] For canine testing, a presentation rate of 33.3 clicks per second has been suggested to obtain quality BAER waves while minimizing testing time for unsedated dogs or puppy screening.[21]

Stimulus intensity Stimulus intensity can have a profound effect on the BAER waveform. In general, absolute BAER wave latencies decrease and amplitudes increase with an increase in stimulus intensity, but interpeak latencies remain more stable.

In human audiology, the intensity of the click stimulus is commonly reported in terms of decibels above the behavioral threshold of a group of normal listeners, referred to as *nHL*.[5,12,22,23] The normal human hearing level for a click stimulus is considered 0 dB nHL.[3] However, these dB nHL values are of questionable use in testing dogs.

Although the dB nHL values observed for the click stimulus in humans are likely similar to what might be seen in dogs, this has not yet been established in the literature. Thus, the correct reference for the intensity of the click stimulus levels should be the actual peak equivalent sound pressure being generated by the click stimulus.[22] The peSPL is the maximum absolute value of the instantaneous sound pressure in the click interval.[3,22] The default intensity of most commercially available systems is in nHL; changing to peSPL only requires going into the menu and clicking on stimulus and selecting "SPL." Using peSPL units to define the stimulus intensities for generating the BAER provides a standardized method of reviewing the results and prevents confusion when comparing data among studies. The reference for 0 dB peak sound pressure is 20 μPa.[3] For any sound, this reference is equal to 20 times the logarithm to the base 10 of the ratio of the pressure of the sound measured to the reference pressure; the typical reference for 0 dB root mean square sound pressure level (SPL) is 20 μPa.[3,14]

Transducers Transducers used to record BAERs in the dog include the insert earphone, standard earphones (ie, headset), and bone conductors. If the transducer used for the BAER test is an insert earphone placed into the external ear canal of the subject, stimulus artifact is reduced relative to stimulus delivery through standard earphones. Compared with standard earphone, insert earphones are comfortable, prevent ear canal collapse, and decrease background noise.[2,3,19] The plastic stimulus delivery tube connected to the insert earphone produces an acoustic time delay of 0.9 ms that must be corrected for in the associated BAER to avoid erroneous prolongation of latency values.[2,3]

Bone-conduction stimulation is used to activate the cochlea via a vibrator. In humans, bone-conduction stimulation may be made through placing the vibration unit either on the mastoid process of the temporal bone or the frontal bone of the head.[3] The headset used in humans for bone-conduction stimulation can be modified for use in the dog through removing the vibration unit from the headset and placing it directly on the mastoid process of the tested ear and holding it in place by hand.[24]

Patient Preparation

Because the BAER is not markedly altered by anesthesia, chemical restraint can be used to obtain these recording. Sedation or anesthesia will allow longer testing times. Once sedated or anesthetized, the animal is placed in sternal recumbency and the head is slightly elevated. In some instances, such as in screening for congenital hearing loss or when shorter testing times are anticipated, the BAER test can be performed on the awake puppy or dog. In these cases, to prevent pain or discomfort, topical anesthetic cream, 2.5% lidocaine and 2.5% prilocaine cream (eutectic mixture of local anesthetics, or EMLA, cream), may be applied to the skin at least 15 minutes before electrode placement.

Rapid-pull 13-mm subdermal needle electrodes are inserted into 3 different locations on the dog, referred to as the *electrical montage*, with the positive, noninverting, electrode placed at the vertex (Cz), located at midline of the subject's head. The negative or inverting electrode is placed just forward of the tragus (A1) of the ear to be tested, and the ground electrode is placed at the nontest ear tragus (A2). This placement is in accordance with the International 10–20 nomenclature, an internationally recognized guide for electrode placements for electroencephalogram and electrophysiologic testing. BAER recordings are obtained between electrodes at the vertex and test ear, which receives the acoustic stimulus, with the opposing ear electrode used as the ground. This placement is then reversed to test the other ear.

Needle electrodes are an important acquisition parameter that conduct bioelectrical activity from the body via wire leads to the recording equipment.[2,25] Needle electrodes provide rapid, secure, and consistent placement when recording BAERs, and allow improved impedance in subjects with fur. The electrodes are attached to a transmitter box, which contains an electrode impedance meter. Electrode impedance is the measure of resistance that an electrical circuit presents to the passage of a current when a voltage is applied.[3,5] In the BAER, electrode impedance is impacted by the surface area, electrode type, and tissue where the electrodes contact the subject. Needle electrodes are preferred for BAERs because the electrode makes more direct electrical contact under the skin surface, lowering impedance.[5] The impedance should be equal between electrodes and be 5000 Ω or less for each electrode to minimize background interference that may affect recording quality and increase recording time.[1,5] The Cz, A1, A2 electrode configuration is considered the most optimal for use by many auditory neurophysiologists because it records auditory nerve and brainstem components concurrently while being less impacted by physiologic noise compared with other electrode configurations.[3,5,6,14,17,19]

Electrode configuration is important because electrode orientation exerts a prominent effect on waveform morphology that impacts the amplitude and latency of the response.[3] When electrode impedance is high or the ground electrode is not adequately connected during testing, the BAER waveform quality will deteriorate because of the electrically noisy test condition.[3] Changes in electrode configuration or incorrect electrode assignment, such as stimulation of the wrong ear or analysis of the wrong electrode combination, can result in the erroneous conclusion that the BAER is absent when it is in fact normal, or can result in incorrectly inverted waveforms.[3,19]

Recording

Air-conducted clicks

Either earphones are inserted one into each ear canal or standard earphones are placed on the ears taking care not to collapse the ear canals. During BAER testing, the auditory click stimulus produced by the computer is presented into one ear canal of the animal by the earphone and recorded by the electrode montage placed on the animal's head. BAERs are generally acquired using a 100-μs broadband click stimulus with 12,000-Hz bandwidth power spectra as tested by sound analysis software. Five stimulus intensities are recommended by the authors for use in diagnostic cases: 70 dB peSPL, 80 dB peSPL, 90 dB peSPL 102 dB peSPL, and 116 dB peSPL. Anything higher than 116 dB peSPL is too high and anything lower than 70 dB peSPL just adds additional time and is only needed if threshold function is being estimated. The stimuli are presented from the lowest level, 70 dB peSPL, sequentially to the highest, 116 peSPL. The scalp electrode configuration records electrical changes in brain activity from activation of the cochlea and brainstem auditory nuclei. This recorded brain activity occurring in the first 10 ms after the stimulus presentation consists of time-locked positive and negative deflections, or waves, recorded by the computer as (up to) 7 resultant waves or peaks.[1,3,6,20] To distinguish the low-amplitude response of the BAER from higher amplitude background noise, a minimum of 1000 to 2000 responses or sweeps should be averaged together to obtain acceptable results.[5,23,26] A minimum of 2 sets of BAER waveforms are required at each stimulus intensity level to establish acceptable replication criteria, defined as each subject having an identifiable wave V peak and/or trough within 0.1 ms across the 2 tracings.[26] An alternating stimulus polarity is commonly used, but rarefaction or condensation stimuli are acceptable.

Tone-pip/tone-burst stimuli

Tone pips/tone bursts may be used to estimate auditory sensitivity for specific frequencies. This test is run similarly to that for click stimuli except "tone burst" must be selected instead of "click," and the frequency of interest (500, 1000, 2000, 4000, or 8000 Hz) must be selected as per equipment guidelines. Alternating polarity is commonly used.[27,28]

Bone-conducted click stimuli

Bone-conduction stimulation may be used to estimate auditory sensitivity for determining conductive losses in hearing and differentiation of sensorineural versus conductive or mixed hearing loss. The external and middle ears are bypassed with this test. This test is run similarly to that for click stimuli except "bone conduction" must be selected instead of "click," and the bone stimulator versus earphone stimulus generator must be selected as per equipment guidelines. Peak differentiation has been shown to be best using condensation polarity, although alternating polarity may result in the least stimulus artifact.[24]

WAVE IDENTIFICATION AND ANALYSIS

Evaluation of the BAER includes the following assessments:

- Wave morphology
- Waveform repeatability
- Absolute wave latencies and wave amplitudes
- Interwave latencies
- Interaural comparisons

The morphology of the BAER waveform is the pattern or overall shape of the waves (see **Fig. 1**).[3,5] BAER wave morphology remains a subjective analysis parameter. Morphology is assessed based on the presence of 4 to 5 vertex positive peaks and the large trough after the fifth vertex positive peak. The fourth and fifth waves in the sequence will occasionally merge into a single broad wave, making identification of all 5 waves impossible. The second wave in the sequence (eg, wave II) is often of sufficiently small amplitude that it is masked by the background recording noise and therefore not readily identifiable.[3,20] Noted variances in the morphology of BAER recordings are not considered unusual and likely result from an interaction among the selected electrode placement sites, acquisition parameters, and electrical transmission characteristics of the various tissues interposed between the neural generators and the electrode recording site.[3]

In keeping with human guidelines and past research on canine BAERs, waves are labeled based on repeatability of the peaks and a comparison of the waveform at the 5 stimulus intensities (70 dB peSPL, 80 dB peSPL, 90 dB peSPL, 102 dB peSPL, and 116 dB peSPL) to verify that peaks were true peaks and not artifact.[3] The stimuli are presented from the lowest level, 70 dB peSPL, sequentially to the highest, 116 peSPL. A typical prerequisite for waveform analysis is repeatability, wherein at least 2 BAER waveforms, recorded in succession with the same stimulus and acquisition measurement conditions, have consistent latency and amplitude measures.[3,15] The absence of replicable waveforms is often an indication of a severe to profound hearing impairment or technical problems, such as inadequate stimulus, improper electrode pairs, or excessive noise artifact.[3]

The latency of each wave is defined as time from the stimulus onset to the positive or negative peak of each wave.[29–31] Wave I is the first positive peak evoked and appears at a latency of approximately 1 to 2 ms, with each subsequent peak occurring at less than 1-ms intervals.[31] The trough of wave V is used as the appropriate indicator of wave V (at the proper approximate latency of 0.48–0.56 ms) relative to the peak of wave V. Wave amplitudes range from less than 1 to 6 µV.[31] Interpeak latency can be measured between any wave pair, but those most commonly measured are between waves I through III and waves I through V (see **Fig. 1**).

When comparing BAER canine data, the click levels used for testing are important given that as stimulus intensity is decreased, the absolute latency of BAER waves increases.[3,5,12,14,20] The higher frequency stimuli elicit shorter latencies than lower frequency stimuli because high frequencies stimulate the more basal portions of the basilar membrane. This process generates earlier BAER responses, because the traveling wave moves from the base to the apex of the cochlea.[5,14,19] Therefore, the stimulus level used to generate a BAER is a critical variable that influences the resultant latency and amplitude.[3,19]

In addition to analyzing individual wave latencies and interwave latencies, wave V latency-intensity (LI) functions can be graphed. Most BAER testing equipment will have a programmed mechanism for producing a graphic of the wave V LI function. After running BAER tests using at least 3 different stimulus intensities and labeling them as waves I to V, this function will graph the waveforms relative to one another, automatically constructing an LI curve. The expectation is that as stimulus intensity is increased, waves will occur at earlier latencies for a normal ear. A shift of the LI curve or change of the slope may indicate hearing loss; however, the result must be compared with a normal population, and currently there are no universal normative LI function curves in the dog. Prediction of types of hearing loss using LI functions has clinical limitations because of patient variability and the very small intensity increments needed to describe the slope of the function. Still, this has been shown to be a useful tool in the dog when used with standard BAER waveform analysis.[32]

USE OF BAER TESTING IN CANINE HEARING ASSESSMENT
Site of Lesion Diagnostic Test

In humans, conductive lesions affecting the external or middle ear may result in a prolonged wave I; however, interwave latencies I through III and I through V are normal. The LI curve parallels the normal curve, although the curve is shifted to the right. The use of bone-conduction stimulation may be useful for determining conductive hearing losses and differentiating sensorineural versus conductive or mixed hearing loss.

One such use of the bone-conduction BAER test in the dog would be in evaluating a Cavalier King Charles spaniel with suspected PSOM (this disease is discussed in more detail in the article by Cole elsewhere in this issue). Briefly, in this disease, the middle ear cavity is filled with mucus. Through using bone-conduction stimuli, which will bypass the middle ear cavity, one would expect to see a normal response to the BAER test at the stimulus intensity at which the air-conducted BAER is no longer attainable (**Fig. 2**). The slope of the LI curve in the Cavalier King Charles spaniel with PSOM is similar to that in those without PSOM, but the LI curve is shifted to the right.[32]

Sensorineural lesions can affect the BAER depending on the site of the lesion. At low intensities, sensory lesions can delay absolute wave intensities while interwave latencies I through III and I through V remain unchanged, whereas at high intensities, the BAER may seem normal because of recruitment of the hair cells in the cochlea. In complete loss of cochlear function, no identifiable waveforms may be present.

BAER testing may be useful in determining whether lesions exist in the central auditory pathway. Lesions may be diagnosed based on increased interwave latencies or missing waves components but not reliably by altered amplitudes.

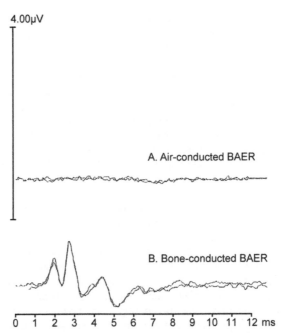

4.00μV

A. Air-conducted BAER

B. Bone-conducted BAER

0 1 2 3 4 5 6 7 8 9 10 11 12 ms

Fig. 2. BAER from the right ear of a 2-year-old Cavalier King Charles spaniel with primary secretory otitis media. A. Air-conducted BAER depicting a flat tracing at 70 dB peSPL. B. Bone-conduction BAER depicting restoration of the BAER waveforms at the same intensity level, confirming conductive hearing loss secondary to the mucus in the middle ear. (*Courtesy of* Dr L.K. Cole and Mr T. Vojt, The Ohio State University, Columbus, OH.)

Estimation of Hearing Threshold

When ABR testing is used to quantify hearing levels, the most commonly used interpretation metric involves identification of the lowest stimulus intensity at which the fifth peak in the sequence, or wave V, can be identified (ie, the wave V threshold). Click stimuli should be delivered at increasing intensities that are no more than 5 dB peSPL apart from one another. The most common method for determining BAER threshold is visual inspection of the averaged waveform.[3,17] A minimum of 2 sets of ABR waveforms are required at each stimulus intensity level to establish acceptable replication criteria (ie, identified wave V peak or trough within 0.1 ms across the 2 tracings).

It is widely recognized in the clinical application of ABR in humans that the wave V threshold measured with click stimuli will be detected at a level within 10 to 15 dB higher or lower than the behavioral pure-tone thresholds in the 2000 to 4000 Hz range. Thresholds estimated from the ABR are typically higher when compared with behavioral thresholds, by as much as 10 to 20 dB depending on frequency. Similarity among dogs is not unexpected.

Screening for Inherited and Pigment-Associated Deafness

According to the Orthopedic Foundation for Animals BAER test examination protocol for puppies, only a single-stimulus intensity between 70 and 105 dB nHL must be run, from which peaks I and V are judged at their appropriate latencies. A puppy showing a repeatable wave V at 70 dB nHL (90 dB peSPL) would be expected to show normal pure-tone thresholds (ie, 15–20 dB HL) in the 2000- to 4000-Hz frequency range.[10]

However, this would be clearly higher than a normal threshold and would therefore mask a mild (or even moderate) hearing loss and be unacceptable in human audiology.

OAES
Background

An OAE is a sound that is generated from within the internal ear. The normal cochlea receives and sends sounds via the external auditory meatus. These sounds are produced directly by the cochlea with the outer hair cells as their source. OAEs were shown experimentally by David Kemp in 1978.[33]

The primary purpose of the OAE test is to determine cochlear (outer hair cell) function. In humans this information is routinely used to screen hearing (particularly in neonates, infants, or individuals with developmental disabilities) and differentiate between the sensory and neural components of sensorineural hearing loss. The patient does not need to attend to the test.

Anatomy and Physiology of OAEs

When sound is used to elicit an OAE, it is sent via the outer ear, where the auditory stimulus is converted from an acoustic signal to a mechanical signal at the tympanic membrane and is transmitted through the middle ear ossicles; the stapes footplate moves in kind at the oval window, causing traveling fluid waves in the cochlea. These traveling waves move the basilar membrane, with each portion of the basilar membrane being sensitive to only a limited-frequency range. The arrangement is tonotopic. In other words, regions closest to the oval window are more sensitive to high-frequency stimuli, whereas regions further away toward the apical end of the basilar membrane are sensitive to low-frequency stimuli. Therefore, for OAEs, the first responses returned and recorded by the probe microphone emanate from the high-frequency cochlear regions. Outer hair cells are located in the organ of Corti on the basilar membrane. These hair cells are motile; an electrochemical response elicits a motor response. The 3 rows of outer hair cells have stereocilia arranged in a W formation. The stereocilia are linked to each other and therefore move as a unit. The outer hair cells are believed to underlie OAE generation.

When the basilar membrane moves, the hair cells are set into motion and an electromechanical response is elicited, producing an afferent and an efferent signal that is emitted back out of the ear canal. This efferent signal is measured in the outer ear canal using OAE equipment.

Recording and Interpretation

OAEs are sounds recorded by a microphone fitted into the ear canal. OAE recordings are made via an ear canal probe that is inserted deeply into the ear canal. Because the test is mechanized, the screening unit will automatically complete the test in discrete stages: determination of noise floor levels (ambient noise), delivery of the signals, and measurement. For the OAE response to be considered a "pass," it must be at least 4 dB SPL higher than the noise floor.

The current issue that confounds most OAE testing in dogs is the ability to get a good seal of the earpiece into the ear canal to obtain an appropriate SNR. The earpiece is not designed for a dog and is uncomfortable enough that most dogs do not tolerate it well when tested awake. However, the test can be performed with the dog sedated or anesthetized.

Auditory testing of OAEs is an effective method for determining the functionality of the cochlea.[34] OAES can be of 2 general types: spontaneous and evoked. Several different cochlear evoked responses can be readily recorded. Evoked OAEs are of specific importance in audiologic assessment. Two types of evoked OAE tests may be used as a test of cochlear function in a clinical setting: transient evoked OAE (TEOAE) and distortion product OAE (DPOAE).

The TEOAE is measured in response to a rapid-onset and a short-duration click stimulus. Most commonly, 80- to 85-dB SPL stimuli are used clinically. TEOAEs are generally recorded over approximately 20 ms. Responses are stored in alternating computer memory banks, A and B. Data that correlate between the 2 memory banks are considered a response. Data that do not correlate are considered noise. This test is commonly used for infant screening,[20] but may also be applied to puppies and dogs (**Fig. 3**).[35–37]

DPOAEs also can be measured in puppies and dogs (**Fig. 4**).[1,35,38] Unlike the TEOAE, the DPOAE is generated by 2 tones (denoted as f_1 and f_2) recorded at a frequency of $2f_1-f_2$, known as the *cubic distortion tone* at 2 intensity levels denoted L1 and L2. A setting of 65/55 dB SPL L1/L2 is frequently used.

Although either OAE technique can be used in animal audiology practice, they are only now being tested for routine clinical use.

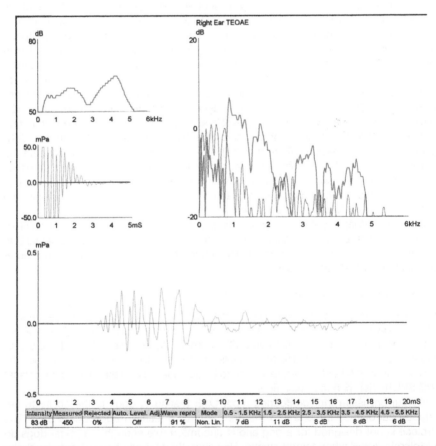

Fig. 3. TEOAE from a normal-hearing Border Collie, right ear, age 8 years. The lower image is the response waveform. For the TEOAE response to be considered a "pass," the SNR must be at least 4 dB sound pressure level for each frequency range. For example, for 1.5 to 2.5 kHz, the SNR ratio is 7 dB. (*Courtesy of* Dr P.M. Scheifele, University of Cincinnati, Cincinnati, OH.)

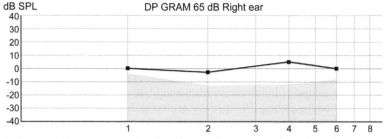

f2	DP	L1	L2	DP level	Noise level	S/N level	Measured	Rejected
1000 Hz	638 Hz	65 dB	55 dB	0.3 dB	-4.9 dB	5.2 dB	74	17%
2000 Hz	1278 Hz	65 dB	55 dB	-3.2 dB	-13.2 dB	10.0 dB	70	19%
4000 Hz	2556 Hz	65 dB	55 dB	5.0 dB	-12.0 dB	17.0 dB	28	0%
6000 Hz	3836 Hz	65 dB	55 dB	0.4 dB	-8.5 dB	8.9 dB	55	2%

S/N stop criteria	Rejection level	Stimulus tolerance	Test time
7 dB	20 dB	± 5 dB	0 min. 48 sec.

Fig. 4. DPOAE from a normal-hearing Border Collie, right ear, age 8 years. For the DPOAE response to be considered a "pass," the S/N must be at least 4 dB sound pressure level for each frequency. The y axis represents frequency in kHz. S/N, signal to noise ratio. (*Courtesy of* Mr T. Vojt, College of Veterinary Medicine, The Ohio State University, Columbus, OH; and Dr P.M. Scheifele, University of Cincinnati, Cincinnati, OH.)

OAE TESTING COMBINED WITH BAER TESTING FOR COMPLETE AUDITORY CLINICAL ASSESSMENT

OAE testing is routinely used in human audiology, especially in combination with ABR testing.[3,5] This test may be used by the audiologist to determine the functionality of the cochlea before conducting central auditory testing (BAER testing). The absence of OAE may indicate hearing loss (outer hair cell damage). It may also indicate outer/middle ear problems, because for a normal OAE transmission to occur, nearly normal outer and middle ear function is required. If the otoscopic check and tympanometry are normal, then a failed OAE test indicates cochlear dysfunction. TEOAE is absent when the hearing loss is around 53 dB peSPL or greater. DPOAE is absent when the hearing loss is around 68 dB peSPL or greater. Thus, the absence of an OAE indicates elevated hearing thresholds.

In human audiology, when used in conjunction with ABR testing, OAEs may be a more accurate method for hearing screening. ABR waveforms may exist when OAEs are absent, because suprathreshold intensities will most certainly activate the inner hair cells and can elicit ABRs. Complete loss of outer hair cells and subsequent loss of OAEs leads to approximately 40 dB of hearing loss. Therefore, a click presented at higher than that level will still yield an ABR. The absence of OAEs and the ABR would indicate profound hearing loss affecting all portions of the cochlea, both the inner and outer hair cells. However, auditory neuropathy, a disease seen in humans but not yet identified in the dog, is typically characterized by normal outer hair cell functions reflected by good OAEs, but abnormal to absent ABRs. The OAE is a rapid test that may be more useful in veterinary hearing screening in the future when used in conjunction with BAER testing.

OVERVIEW OF THE ASSR

ASSRs are electrophysiologic responses of the brain that result from the amplitude and frequency characteristics of an amplitude- or frequency-modulated stimulus. The

ASSR response is steady in both amplitude and phase relative to that stimulus.[2] Modulated stimuli that change over time induce responses from the brain that occur in coincidence with the modulation pattern. These responses are known as the "following responses." For example, a 4000-Hz tone amplitude modulated 50% at 70 Hz will go from 100% amplitude to 50% and back to 100% 70 times per second. The frequency content of a modulated (varied periodic wave, the carrier signal) stimulus tone can elicit the change of response of the brain or "frequency-following response" in synchrony with the modulation frequency (70 Hz in the example). But for the brain to be able to react to the modulation frequency, the cochlea must be sensitive to the carrier signal (4000 Hz in the example). If the cochlea is not sensitive to the 4000-Hz signal at the given intensity level, the ASSR will be absent. The ASSR is essentially a statistical estimation of whether a threshold is present based on the assumption that the related neural responses coincide with the stimulus repetition rate.[2] The phase delay of the ASSR response is analogous to the latency of waves in an ABR/BAER.[39,40]

Because the ASSR is based on statistical measures, it does not require interpretation of waveforms and hence is a more objective measure.[40] In addition, the ASSR can allow for estimation of frequency-specific hearing thresholds and the testing of multiple frequencies (carrier frequencies of 500, 1000, 2000, and 4000 Hz typically) in both ears simultaneously, thereby shortening test time.[39] An example of an ASSR output is shown in **Fig. 5.**

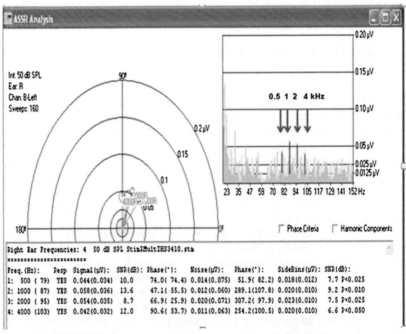

Fig. 5. Typical ASSR analysis output for a normal hearing adult. Stimulus frequencies were 0.5, 1.0, 2.0, and 4.0 kHz with modulation frequencies of 79, 85, 93, and 203 Hz, respectively. The upper right panel shows synchronized activity of the ASSR (*highlighted in red*) at each of the 4 modulation frequencies along with their corresponding carrier frequencies. The polar plot shows the response phases of the 4 ASSR responses to the 4 modulation stimuli. (*From* Balvalli SN, Stephens J, Scott M, et al. Comparison of behavioral and auditory steady state response thresholds using a sound-field stimulus in cochlear implant recipients. Mentored Doctoral Poster at the 13th Symposium on Cochlear Implants in Children. Chicago, Illinois, July 14-16, 2011; with permission.)

The same electrode montage (International 10–20) used for ABR recordings is used for the ASSR. The stimulus is delivered through insert earphones, headphones, a bone oscillator, or a free field (through speakers) as they would be for ABR/BAER testing. An overview comparison of some primary differences between ASSR and BAER are as follows:

- ASSR is induced using a repetitive sound stimulus presented at a high rate, whereas BAER uses a transient (click) sound produced at a low rate.
- ASSR enables the evaluation of frequency-specific information binaurally and more rapidly than BAER.
- ASSR analysis relates to amplitude and phases in the frequency spectrum, whereas BAER is relative to amplitude and latency.
- ASSR uses a statistical analysis methodology accurate to 91% to 95% confidence, whereas BAER depends highly on a subjective analysis of the amplitude/latency function and waveform morphology.

A drawback to ASSR is that the dog must be still to obtain accurate and reliable results. In this sense the ASSR is currently more unforgiving than BAER testing for dogs. Still, the ASSR holds future promise as a method for rapid and accurate assessment of hearing acuity in animals.[41]

SUMMARY

Given the high incidence of deafness within several breeds of dogs and the concerns owners have when their pet's hearing begins to diminish with presbycusis (age-related hearing loss), accurate hearing screening and assessment of canine hearing is essential. In addition to the BAER test, 2 other electrophysiologic tests are now being examined as audiologic tools for use in veterinary medicine: OAEs and the ASSR.

BAER testing has long been used routinely in veterinary practice to screen breeds that are commonly afflicted with congenital deafness, demonstrate normal hearing thresholds for working and service dogs to determine whether they can respond appropriately to environmental auditory cues, detect presbycusis, diagnose ear pathologies such as PSOM, and identify progressive or acquired hearing impairments to long-term noise exposure (eg, kennel noise) or repeated, sudden-intense impact noise exposure. Just as in human ABR testing, to improve the BAER testing of animals and ensure an accurate interpretation of test findings from one test site to another, the establishment of and adherence to clear protocols is essential, which includes standardized click presentation rate and bandwidth filter settings and the use of peSPL in place of an nHL.

OAEs assess the functionality of the outer hair cells within the cochlea, although the absence of OAEs sheds little light on the actual degree of cochlear hearing loss. Regardless, this rapid test may eventually prove to be of great clinical utility in veterinary hearing screening and diagnostic assessment if used with BAER.

The ASSR is not used in screening but rather when a more comprehensive hearing assessment is needed. The ASSR holds promise as an objective modality for rapid testing of multiple frequencies in both ears simultaneously. As such, the ASSR allows canine hearing evaluation to be completed more efficiently than the BAER.

REFERENCES

1. Strain GM. Brainstem auditory evoked response (BAER). In: Deafness in dogs and cats. Cambridge (MA): CABI; 2011. p. 83–5.

2. Petrak MR. Evaluating hearing in infants and small children. Available at: http://www.audiologyonline.com/articles/article_detail.asp?article_id=242. Accessed September 10, 2011.

3. Hall JW III. New handbook of auditory evoked responses. Boston: Pearson Education Inc; 2007.

4. Jewett DL, Williston JS. Auditory evoked far fields averaged from the scalp of humans. Brain 1971;4:681–96.

5. Musiek FE, Rintelmann WF. Contemporary perspectives in hearing assessment. Boston: Allyn and Bacon; 1999. p. 197–222.

6. Plourde EG. Auditory evoked potentials. Best Pract Res Clin Anaesthesiol 2006; 20(1):129–39.

7. Legatt AD. Brainstem auditory evoked potentials: methodology, interpretation, and clinical application. In: Aminoff MJ, editor. Electrodiagnosis in clinical neurology. 4th edition. New York: Churchill Livingstone; 1999. p. 451–84.

8. Chiappa KH, Hill RA. Brainstem auditory evoked potentials: interpretation. In: Chiappa KH, editor. Evoked potentials in clinical medicine. 3rd edition. Philadelphia: Lippincott-Raven; 1997. p. 199–249.

9. BAER testing protocol. Orthopedic Foundation for Animals Web site. Available at: http://www.offa.org/deaf_baer.html. Accessed June 4, 2012.

10. Heffner HE. Hearing in large and small dogs: absolute thresholds and size of the tympanic membrane. Behav Neurosci 1983;97(2):310–8.

11. Strain GM. What is the BAER test? Available at: http://www.lsu.edu/deafness/baerexpl.htm. Accessed June 15, 2012.

12. Moller AR. Hearing: its physiology and pathophysiology. Boston: Academic Press; 2000.

13. Dewey CW. Breed-associated neurologic abnormalities of dogs and cats. In: Curtis CW, editor. A practical guide to canine and feline neurology. 2nd edition. Ames (IO): Blackwell Publishing; 2008. p. 4–6.

14. Burkard RF, Don M, Eggermont JJ. Auditory evoked potentials basic principles and clinical applications. Baltimore (MD): Lippincott Williams and Wilkins; 2007.

15. Callison DM. Audiologic evaluation of hearing-impaired infants and children. Otolaryngol Clin North Am 1999;32(6):1009–18.

16. Wilson WJ, Mills PC. Brainstem auditory-evoked response in dogs. Am J Vet Res 2005;66(12):2177–87.

17. Sininger YS. Auditory brain stem response for objective measures of hearing. Ear Hear 1993;14(1):23–30.

18. Guidelines 9a: Guidelines on evoked potentials. American Clinical Neurophysiology Society Web site. Available at: http://www.acns.org. Accessed November 18, 2011.

19. Hood LJ. Stimulus, recording, and patient factors influencing the ABR. In: Danhauer JL, editor. Clinical applications of the auditory brainstem response. Clifton Park (NY): Singular Publishing Group; 1998. p. 12–63.

20. Picton TW. Auditory brainstem responses: peaks along the way. In: Human auditory evoked potentials. San Diego (CA): Plural Publishing; 2011. p. 213–45.

21. Wilson WJ, Mils PC, Bradley AP, et al. Fast assessment of canine hearing using high click-rate BAER. Vet J 2011;187:136–8.

22. Mendel LL, Danhauer JL, Singh S. Singular's illustrated dictionary of audiology. London: Singular; 1999.

23. Holliday TA, Te Selle ME. Brain stem auditory-evoked potentials of dogs: wave forms and effects of recording electrode positions. Am J Vet Res 1985;46(4): 845–51.

24. Strain GM, Green KD, Twedt AC, et al. Brain stem auditory evoked potentials from bone conduction stimulation in dogs. Am J Vet Res 1993;54:1817–21.
25. Marshall AE. Brain stem auditory-evoked response of the nonanesthetized dog. Am J Vet Res 1985;46(4):966–73.
26. Mitchell C, Phillips DS, Trune DR. Variables affecting the auditory brainstem response: audiogram, age, gender, and head size. Hear Res 1989;40(1–2):75–86.
27. Ter Haar G, Venker-van Haagen AJ, de Groot HN, et al. Click and low, middle-, and high-frequency toneburst stimulation of the canine cochlea. J Vet Intern Med 2002;16:274–80.
28. Uzuka Y, Fukaki M, Hara Y, et al. Brainstem auditory evoked responses elicited by tone-burst stimuli in clinically normal dogs. J Vet Intern Med 1998;12:22–5.
29. Munro KJ, Shiu JN, Cox CL. The effect of head size on the auditory brainstem response for two breeds of dog. Br J Audiol 1997;31(5):309–14.
30. Don M, Ponton CW, Eggermont JJ, et al. Gender differences in cochlear response time: an explanation for gender amplitude differences in the unmasked auditory brain-stem response. J Acoust Soc Am 1993;94(4):2135–48.
31. Sims MH. Diseases of the ear canal: electrodiagnostic evaluation of auditory function. Vet Clin North Am Small Anim Pract 1988;18:913–44.
32. Harcourt-Brown TR, Parker JE, Granger N, et al. Effect of middle ear effusion on the brain-stem auditory evoked response of Cavalier King Charles Spaniels. Vet J 2011;188:341–5.
33. Kemp D. Stimulated acoustic emissions from within the human auditory system. J Acoust Soc Am Nov 1978;64(5):1386–91.
34. Robinette MS, Glattke TJ. Otoacoustic emissions: clinical applications. 3rd edition. New York: Thieme; 2007.
35. Sockalingam R, Filippich L, Sommerlad S, et al. Transient-evoked and 2(F1-F2) distortion product otoacoustic emissions in dogs: preliminary findings. Audiol Neurootol 1998;3:373–85.
36. Sims MH, Rogers RK, Thelin JW. Transiently evoked otoacoustic emissions in dogs. Progr Vet Neurol 1994;5:49–56.
37. McBrearty A, Penderis J. Transient evoked otoacoustic emissions testing for screening of sensorineural deafness is puppies. J Vet Intern Med 2011;25:1366–71.
38. Schemera B, Blumsack JT, Cellino AF, et al. Evaluation of otoacoustic emissions in clinically normal alert puppies. Am J Vet Res 2011;72:295–301.
39. John MS, Picton TW. Human auditory steady-state responses to amplitude-modulated tones: phase and latency measurements. J Heart Res 2000;141(1–2):57–9.
40. Rance G. Auditory steady-state response: generation, recording and clinical applications. New York: Plural Publishing; 2008. p. 67-70.
41. Markessis E, Ponselet L, Colin C, et al. Auditory steady-state evoked potentials (ASSEPs): a study of optional stimulation parameters for frequency-specific threshold measurement in dogs. Clin Neurophysiol 2006;117:1760–71.

Ototoxicity in Dogs and Cats

Naoki Oishi, MD[a,b], Andra E. Talaska, BS[c], Jochen Schacht, PhD[c],*

KEYWORDS

- Hearing loss • Cisplatin • Aminoglycosides • Diuretics

KEY POINTS

- Aminoglycosides (eg, gentamicin, amikacin) and cisplatin are the drugs of highest concern for ototoxicity.
- Loss of sensory cells (hair cells) in the internal ear is the primary cause of permanent deficits in hearing or balance.
- Use of compensatory mechanisms by domestic animals (observation of body language with spoken commands or visual cues to aid balance) may obscure or delay the detection of sensory deficits.

INTRODUCTION

The awareness that therapeutic treatments sometimes impose undesirable side effects ranging from minor inconveniences to death is as ancient as the practice itself of treating ailments with herbs and drugs. In particular, the knowledge that some agents have the potential to adversely affect the senses of hearing and balance has a history going back at least a thousand years.[1] It is notable that these side effects were all first discovered in humans, including the landmark discoveries of auditory and vestibular toxicity (ototoxicity) of aminoglycoside antibiotics and cisplatin in the twentieth century. Only subsequently did laboratory experiments establish animal models from which further insight into toxic mechanisms was gained and which can be used to delineate safe or protective treatments.

A surprisingly wide variety of drugs are potentially ototoxic, varying in chemical structure and therapeutic targets (**Table 1**). In human medicine, the list includes drugs

Dr Schacht's research on ototoxicity is supported by grant no. DC-003685 from the National Institutes on Deafness and Other Communication Disorders, National Institutes of Health. The authors declare no conflicts of interest.
[a] Kresge Hearing Research Institute, Department of Otolaryngology, University of Michigan Medical School, Medical Sciences Building I, 1150 West Medical Center Drive, Ann Arbor, MI 48109–5616, USA; [b] Department of Otolaryngology, Keio University School of Medicine, 35 Shinanomachi, Shinjuku, Tokyo 160-8582, Japan; [c] Kresge Hearing Research Institute, Department of Otolaryngology, University of Michigan Medical School, Room 5315, Medical Sciences Building I, 1150 West Medical Center Drive, Ann Arbor, MI 48109–5616, USA
* Corresponding author.
E-mail address: Schacht@umich.edu

Vet Clin Small Anim 42 (2012) 1259–1271
http://dx.doi.org/10.1016/j.cvsm.2012.08.005
0195-5616/12/$ – see front matter

Table 1 Potential causes of hearing loss	
Aminoglycoside antibiotics	Streptomycin, neomycin, gentamicin
Antineoplastics	Cisplatin, carboplatin
Diuretics	Ethacrynic acid, furosemide
Metallo compounds	Arsenicals, mercurials
Antimalarial	Quinine
Analgesics, antipyretics	Salicylates
Polypeptide antibiotics	Viomycin, vancomycin
Macrolide antibiotics	Erythromycin
Industrial solvents	Toluene, organotins
Environment	Noise, age

The table lists representatives of potentially ototoxic agents and environmental causes of hearing loss. Information is derived from literature on experimental animals and clinical data.[8] The compilation is intended to show the range of drugs and environmental factors that can affect the auditory (and to some extent the vestibular) system in mammals. As further outlined in the text and in **Table 2** the effects of the various agents may be transient or permanent and the incidence of such effects can be highly variable.

of past interest (eg, arsenicals, mercurials); drugs that only cause a temporary effect on hearing (eg, salicylates); and drugs in current use associated with a significant incidence of permanent hearing loss (aminoglycosides, cisplatin). Of potential concern in veterinary practice are primarily the antibacterial aminoglycoside antibiotics gentamicin and amikacin, the anticancer agent cisplatin, and loop diuretics, such as furosemide, all of which are discussed in this article. Some ototoxic potential might also be associated with occasionally or rarely used drugs, such as the anthelmintic arsenical melarsomine and the antibiotic erythromycin. It is of interest to note that some of these therapeutics also exhibit renal toxicity, as has been documented for aminoglycosides and cisplatin, and some nonsteroidal anti-inflammatory agents. Finally, in considering potential causes of hearing loss in animals, environmental factors should not be overlooked, such as advanced age and even exposure to noise in large kennels.[2]

OTOTOXICITY IN DOGS AND CATS

The incidence of therapy-linked ototoxicity in domestic dogs and cats is difficult, perhaps impossible, to establish. Subtle changes in hearing go largely unnoticed by pet owners because these animals either rely more on or compensate with their other senses. Verbal commands are frequently accompanied by body language that helps their interpretation in the presence of a compromised hearing, and visual cues and some inherent plasticity of the vestibular system hide small effects on balance. As a result, animals with auditory or vestibular deficits may function reasonably well in a familiar environment, an adaptation that is likewise observed in humans. However, with increasing duration of chemotherapy as might be needed for cancer or with confounding factors, such as aging, the impediments can become so severe as to affect gait and balance or even be a risk to life if an approaching danger, such as a car, cannot be heard. This article addresses the potential ototoxicity of cisplatin, gentamicin, furosemide, and related compounds, drawing from laboratory animal studies and human clinical trials, which have been well documented over decades of research and experience.

GENTAMICIN

Gentamicin is one of the aminoglycosides, a class of antibiotics that is effective mainly against gram-negative bacteria. Since the discovery of the first aminoglycoside (strep-tomycin) in 1944[3] and, subsequently, other compounds of this class (gentamicin in 1963),[4] they have been widely popular because of their broad antibacterial spectrum, nonallergenic characteristics, and inexpensive cost. In cats and dogs these drugs are primarily used to treat septicemia and infections of bone, joints, the respiratory tract, skin, soft tissue, urinary tract, and uterus, and are given topically for ear infections. Aminoglycosides generally are administered systemically (intravenously, intramuscu-larly, or subcutaneously) or topically into the ear, and all routes of administration have the potential to lead to ototoxic side effects. They are ineffective given orally because they are not absorbed enterically.

Although the antibacterial action is complex, a major contributing mechanism seems to be an inhibition of protein synthesis accomplished through binding to the bacterial 30S small ribosomal subunit.[5] Because of their long history as therapeutics and sometimes uncontrolled use, bacterial resistance to aminoglycosides has been developing worldwide, not only in human hosts, but also in their veterinary applica-tions.[6] Nevertheless, they still serve as potent antibacterial agents and their judicious use can minimize the further development of resistance.

Incidence of Ototoxicity

Because bacterial ribosomes, the therapeutic targets of aminoglycosides, differ struc-turally from mammalian ones, the drug action is largely specific for prokaryotes. However, mammalian mitochondrial RNA contains similar subunits and may represent a potential target for aminoglycoside antibiotics. In humans, mitochondrial mutations are a well-defined high-risk factor in aminoglycoside-induced hearing loss.[7] To the best of our knowledge, no such risk factors have been identified in domestic animals.

The pattern of ototoxicity differs among the various aminoglycosides, involving either the auditory system (cochleotoxicity) or vestibular system (vestibulotoxicity), or both, but across the board the deficits are typically bilateral, progressive, and essentially inevitable with long-term administration. Gentamicin targets both senses, often with a predilection for balance; amikacin, in contrast, may preferentially target the cochlea.[8] Although a large body of information on ototoxicity in animals exists, the incidence of drug-induced hearing loss cannot be deduced because the goal of laboratory studies is to achieve ototoxicity with high-dose regimens to investigate mechanisms of cell death or prevention. In clinical studies, the reported incidence varies because of differing treatment regimens and, chiefly, varying assessment parameters and definitions of hearing loss. The estimated incidence of ototoxicity in humans, including cochleotoxicity and vestibulotoxicity, ranges from 15% to 50%[9-11] but such data include all measurable hearing and balance deficits and are not indicative of disabling conditions. Aminoglycosides may also cause nephrotoxi-city, but there is no statistically significant relationship to ototoxicity and the incidence of co-occurrence is only 4.5%.[12]

Observation of cats in veterinary treatment confirms the potential for ototoxicity in this species. When renal failure, a frequent side effect of aminoglycoside antibiotics, was diagnosed in cats receiving paromomycin for treatment of infectious enteritis the authors also noticed deafness in three of those four cats.[13] They attributed it to an "excessive dosage" of the drug confounded by renal failure. Apramycin, mostly used in livestock, was tested in a small number of dogs and cats as part of a toxicity assessment. Chronic oral administration to beagle dogs produced little or no signs of nephrotoxicity or ototoxicity probably because of poor absorption after oral dosing. Subcutaneous injections into cats (20% aqueous solution for 30 days) caused severe nephrotoxicity but a possible vestibular problem in only one of the four animals.[14] Clearly, the type of aminoglycoside and the route of administration can influence the nature and incidence of adverse side effects.

Of special concern is that the aminoglycoside antibiotics can cross the placental barrier and, thus, have the potential to cause deafness in the fetus. Experimental studies in rats, mice, guinea pigs, and cats have confirmed the existence of a "critical period" in development when sensitivity to ototoxic agents is greatest.[15–17] This critical period coincides with the development of the inner ear in altricial and precocial mammals.[18]

Internal Ear Pathology

Although various types of cells in the internal ear are affected by long-term administration of aminoglycosides, the sensory cells, predominantly the outer hair cells (OHC), are the primary target of the drugs (**Table 2**). These nonregenerative OHCs begin to die off in the basal region of the cochlear spiral and losses progress toward the middle and apical turns as the lesions worsen. This corresponds with the clinical and experimental observations of initial deterioration of hearing at higher frequencies, which are processed in the basal turn.[19] Such a primary effect on high frequencies might be particularly disturbing for such animals as dogs, which possess hearing at ultrahigh tones. However, prolonged treatment or high doses of drugs increasingly affect lower frequencies and impact the animal (and human) communication range. Other structures in the internal ear are affected later, including the stria vascularis, the structure essential to maintain cochlear homeostasis, and the spiral ganglion cells of the nerve connection to the brain. Although loss of hair cells is the primary reason for the decline of hearing function, all of these pathologic changes are contributing factors and have been observed in cats and dogs.[20,21]

Aminoglycoside antibiotics are also able to produce vestibular lesions and consequent behavioral deficits. Impaired balance is similarly caused by loss of the sensory hair cells of the vestibule, primarily type I hair cells, followed by type II hair cells. The

Table 2
Effects of ototoxins on the internal ear

	Aminoglycosides	Cisplatin	Furosemide
Type of hearing loss	Usually permanent	Usually permanent	Usually temporary
Frequency range of hearing loss	High frequencies with progression to lower frequencies	High frequencies with progression to lower frequencies	Middle frequencies
Hair cell loss	Beginning in the base and progressing toward the apex	Beginning in the base and progressing toward the apex	None
Changes in the stria vascularis	Gross degeneration only at later stages of intoxication	Generally observed; mostly in intermediate cells	Temporary effects on intermediate cells and strial edema
Changes in the cochlear nerve	Nerve degeneration after hair cell loss	Damage at the basal coil, and decrease in function	Temporary impairment of function
Side effects on balance	Possibly severe with some but not all aminoglycosides	Not expected	Not expected

cells are first lost in the apex of the cristae ampullares, the structure responsible for the detection of angular acceleration and deceleration.[22] Damage may also involve the striolar regions of the maculae in utricle and sacculus. Early studies attest that cats can be affected by the vestibular side effects of aminoglycosides,[23,24] but these were laboratory experiments using high doses of the drugs. Such studies indicate the potential toxicity but cannot predict an incidence of vestibulotoxicity in a normal veterinary treatment.

Molecular Mechanisms

Oxidative stress caused by the overproduction of reactive oxygen species (ROS) is implicated in aminoglycoside ototoxicity by many reports.[25–27] ROS, or free radicals, are normal by-products of metabolism and contained by the cells' complement of anti-oxidants. Their excessive formation, however, triggers several well-defined pathways of cell death in the affected cells, including caspase activation and the c-Jun N-terminal kinase/mitogen-activated protein kinase pathway, and caspase-independent apoptotic and necrotic pathways.[28]

Prevention of Ototoxicity

The formation of ROS and subsequent cell death in the cochlea are successfully prevented by the coadministration of antioxidants or similar scavengers of ROS. The efficacy of such cotreatment has been well established in laboratory studies in several species where, for example, gentamicin-induced ototoxicity could be reduced morphologically (prevention of hair cell loss) and functionally (attenuation of hearing impairment).[29] The list of beneficial antioxidants includes deferoxamine and dihydroxybenzoic acid (as iron chelators they prevent the "Fenton-reaction" of ROS formation); glutathione; α-lipoic acid; D-methionine; N-acetylcysteine; herbal preparations (eg, Salviae miltiorrhizae extract); and many more. A randomized double-blind placebo-controlled clinical trial extended the observation of therapeutic protection to patients receiving gentamicin for acute infection. Aspirin, given for its iron-chelating and antioxidant properties, significantly reduced the incidence of gentamicin-induced hearing loss, from 13% (14 of 106 patients) in the placebo group to only 3% (3 of 89) in the aspirin group.[30] These experimental and clinical results strongly support the notion that the formation of ROS causally relates to cell death pathways in aminoglycoside ototoxicity and that antioxidants are potent antidotes.

Despite such progress in prevention, there is presently no guideline for protective cotreatments for dogs and cats receiving potentially ototoxic medications. Because the effects of antioxidants on aminoglycoside ototoxicity have proved robust across species, antioxidant supplements might be interesting candidates for veterinary medicine because of their easy availability, safety, and low cost. Extrapolating from laboratory studies, antioxidant treatment might be most efficacious if the patient can be pretreated with the antioxidant and receive cotreatment for the duration of the aminoglycoside's course. To this date, even experimental studies of prevention of ototoxicity in dogs and cats are lacking and it remains uncertain which antioxidants are effective in these species. Aspirin, for example, would have to be ruled out because of its high toxicity to cats. It is very encouraging, however, that the antioxidants silymarin and vitamin E are effective against the renal side effects of gentamicin in dogs.[31]

CISPLATIN

Since its introduction as an antineoplastic agent in the 1960s, cisplatin has been applied broadly to a variety of malignant tumors, including testicular, ovarian, bladder, and head and neck tumors in humans,[32] and is likewise used in veterinary medicine. An early and clinically significant adverse effect of cisplatin is nephrotoxicity, which can cause irreversible damage to the kidney. However, nephrotoxicity can be successfully reduced by adequate pretreatment and posttreatment hydration and concomitant diuresis. Avoidance of the other typical adverse effects of cisplatin, ototoxicity and neurotoxicity, does not yet have any clinically prescribed regimen or prevention, although recommendations are often made to dose slowly over days and weeks to avert toxicities.

The primary effect of cisplatin in cancer cells is to inhibit DNA replication by intercalating with the bases (binding preferably to the 7-nitrogen atom of guanine), and eventually induce cell death by apoptosis.[33] Although cisplatin is generally highly effective, pathways of resistance do exist, including decreased cellular accumulation (reduced uptake); inactivation of cisplatin by glutathione and metallothionein; enzymatic DNA repair; and resistance to apoptosis.

Incidence of Ototoxicity

The pathophysiologic damage from cisplatin ototoxicity is mostly irreversible. The auditory system is affected almost exclusively and cisplatin-induced hearing loss, just like aminoglycoside-induced hearing loss, commences at the high frequencies. The hearing loss is bilaterally progressive and profound. Its severity is cumulatively dose-dependent and may continue to progress after the administration of the drug is completed. In clinical situations, up to 100% of patients may sustain some degree of hearing loss with prolonged treatment.[34] Various species of experimental animals are likewise susceptible to this drug and the incidence of hearing loss generally is high.[35]

Internal Ear Pathology

Although loss of OHCs is a major pathologic feature, the action of cisplatin on the internal ear seems to be more complex than that of the aminoglycosides, affecting a variety of cell types (see **Table 2**). Along with hearing loss at higher frequencies, audiologic findings in cisplatin ototoxicity include reduction of the endocochlear potential,[36] the electrochemical driving force generated by the stria vascularis and necessary for the transduction of the acoustic stimulus into receptor potentials and subsequent nerve impulses to the brain. Elevation of the thresholds for the compound action potential[37,38] and the cochlear microphonic[38,39] imply a compromised function of vestibulocochlear nerve fibers and OHCs, respectively. Indeed, observations from human temporal bones and experimental animals confirm pathologic changes encompassing the organ of Corti, stria vascularis, and spiral ganglion cells. However, the vestibular system is notably unaffected.[37]

Molecular Mechanisms

Just as is the case for aminoglycosides, the excessive production of ROS seems to be central to cisplatin ototoxicity,[40] and an internal ear-specific NADPH oxidase, NOX3, plays an important role in generating those ROS.[41] ROS then initiate a cascade of cell death pathways leading to apoptosis, where several caspases and Bcl-2 family proteins are activated.[42] Success in experimentally ameliorating cisplatin-induced hearing loss by interfering with these signaling pathways supports a causal relationship between the molecular observations and auditory deficits. As a case in point, the inhibition of NOX3 in the rat cochlea led to the protection of the ear from cisplatin ototoxicity.[43,44] Likewise, inhibitors of caspases protected OHCs and preserved hearing function.[45] These results, however, are derived from laboratory studies that have not yet led to clinical application.

Prevention of Ototoxicity

Given an ROS-based mechanism of cisplatin toxicity, antioxidants have been extensively explored as protective agents.[35,46,47] Supplements tested for their efficacy include glutathione, superoxide dismutase, vitamin C, vitamin A, vitamin E, and transferrin. Here again, studies in animal models have had success[47,48] but clinical studies of antioxidant-based amelioration of cisplatin ototoxicity are minimal.[49] Nevertheless, antioxidants are possibly the most commonly used supplements in patients with cancer, thought to treat the cancer directly, and increase immune function and reduce toxicity of cancer chemotherapies. Of specific interest is that antioxidants have been used in veterinary medicine as cancer therapy or adjunct with such medications as cisplatin.[50–52] This treatment is, however, not without caveat. It has been argued that reducing the toxicity with antioxidants may also reduce cisplatin efficacy toward cancer cells and, hence, efficacy of the chemotherapy. The topic is still controversial and under discussion.[53]

DIURETICS

Furosemide is one of the most commonly used loop diuretics, acting on epithelial cells in the loop of Henle of the kidney, and a drug of choice to treat edema and hypertension. Depending on dose and rate of administration, furosemide can cause several side effects. Electrolytic abnormalities, such as hyponatremia and hypokalemia, and dehydration are common because furosemide changes the level of electrolytes in the blood and the body's total fluid volume. In addition, ototoxicity can be a side effect of furosemide that is, in contrast to aminoglycosides and cisplatin, mostly temporary and rarely permanent.[54,55] However, furosemide has the ability to potentiate cisplatin and aminoglycoside-induced hearing loss to the extent that combination treatment may lead to complete deafness even at individually safe doses of the two agents.[56–59] This danger of potentiation is shared with other diuretics (eg, ethacrynic acid). The mechanism behind potentiation is unknown, but the diuretic may increase the concentration of the ototoxins in the cochlear endolymph.

Incidence of Ototoxicity

Little is known about the clinical incidence of ototoxicity of diuretics because most cases of hearing impairment are transient. One study on humans reported that 4 (6.4%) of 62 of those receiving furosemide had at least a 15-dB elevation of pure tone auditory thresholds[60] and hearing losses were greatest in the middle frequencies. It can be expected that the adverse effects depend on the dose and the frequency of administration. Vertigo has only been seen as an infrequent side effect of furosemide therapy.

Internal Ear Pathology

The pathology induced by diuretics differs significantly from aminoglycosides and cisplatin (see **Table 2**). Diuretics, such as furosemide, primarily act on the nonsensory tissues of the internal ear and by mechanisms detectable only by invasive physiologic measurements that elude routine examination in patients. One manifestation, for example, is a decreased endocochlear potential observed in several animal species, including the dog and the cat.[61,62] Furosemide also reduced the amplitude of the vestibulocochlear nerve action potential in the cat and the dog.[60,63,64] The cochlear microphonic is also affected.[65,66] Corresponding to those functional changes, edema in the stria vascularis and degeneration of intermediate cells of the stria vascularis were observed in guinea pigs.[67] The same kind of morphologic change was reported in a study of a human temporal bone.[68] All of these changes are generally reversible and no permanent morphologic damage to hair cells has been found.

As with aminoglycoside antibiotics, animals in their developmental period are more susceptible to furosemide. Young rat pups have significantly greater reductions in endocochlear potential after diuretic treatment and higher elevation of compound action potential thresholds than rats older than 30 days.[69] The observed physiologic changes were accompanied by edema of the stria vascularis. To what extent other animal species are susceptible has not yet been explored.

Molecular Mechanisms

The molecular mechanism of ototoxicity of diuretics seems closely related to their pharmacologic properties. The kidney and the internal ear have extensive ion-transporting epithelia that are targeted. Consistent with such a mechanism, treatment of guinea pigs with furosemide caused an increase in the sodium concentration and a reduction in potassium activity in the endolymph.[70] This effect may occur by a blockade of active potassium transport in the stria vascularis and is in accordance with the documented decrease of the endocochlear potential.

Prevention of Ototoxicity

Because of the numerous distinctions between the pathologies of furosemide ototoxicity and that of cisplatin and aminoglycosides, antioxidant therapy cannot be assumed to be effective against furosemide ototoxicity. Several other agents, however, have been shown to attenuate the ototoxicity of diuretics: inhalation of oxygen, coadministration of triamterene (a potassium-sparing diuretic), iodinated benzoic acid derivatives (diatrizoate and probenecid), and organic acids (sodium salicylate and penicillin G) provided some protection.[60,71] Overall, however, pharmacologic intervention is of little clinical concern because the ototoxicity of diuretics is usually transient.

SUMMARY

Although little direct data exist on the ototoxicity of drugs in cats and dogs, information from laboratory animals and human patients suggests that domestic animals are similarly susceptible to the major causative agents cisplatin, aminoglycosides, and diuretics. Initial signs of aminoglycoside-induced hearing loss (gentamicin, amikacin) in dogs and cats are difficult to assess in daily life. Standard acoustic "startle tests" (clapping hands behind an animal's back) might be helpful, but are not very sensitive. Alternatively, signs of vestibular dysfunction, such as vomiting, and disturbance of gait in severe lesions may be easier to detect. Initial indications of cisplatin-induced hearing loss may likewise not be apparent in daily activities. Signs of vestibular dysfunction are unlikely because of the drug's preferential action on the auditory system. If initial audiologic deficits from cisplatin (or aminoglycosides) remain unnoticed and the drug continues to be administered, the animals can be expected to develop severe hearing loss.

Administration of aminoglycosides to pregnant dogs or cats may lead to hearing deficits in their offspring. Because most cases of diuretic-induced ototoxicity are only transient, close attention to the dose and rate of injection may avert permanent damage to the inner ear. Newborn or older animals are at greater risk for ototoxicity.

Combination of diuretics with aminoglycoside antibiotics or cisplatin in experimental animals and in humans potentiates for profound, permanent hearing loss. It is possible that ototoxicity in general can be averted by monitoring of hearing and balance and early cessation of treatment or substitution of different drugs. Supplementation of various antioxidants has been demonstrated to attenuate ototoxicity induced by aminoglycosides and, to some extent, cisplatin. Guidelines for palliative treatment of cats and dogs are not yet available.

GLOSSARY

This glossary does not provide complete anatomic or physiologic information but is intended to convey the meaning or interpretation of technical terms. Additional information can be found in other articles in this issue.

Auditory thresholds. The lowest sound intensity that evokes a "hearing" sensation. In animals it is generally measured by auditory brainstem evoked responses, which are recorded noninvasively as a train of electrical waves that travel along the auditory pathway. Auditory thresholds obtained in this fashion are an objective and sensitive determinant of hearing acuity or hearing loss.

Cochlear microphonic. A sound-evoked electrical potential that originates in the outer hair cells and can be taken as an indicator of their proper function.

Compound action potential. This reflects the activity of hair cells and the action potentials of the auditory afferent nerves and thereby provides information on the normal or abnormal processing of sound in the cochlea.

Cristae ampullares, sacculus, utricle. These are individual structures of the vestibular system that adjust one's balance to angular or linear acceleration and gravitational pull. The **macula** is the sensory part of the sacculus and the utricle, containing hair cells; the **striola** is a central segment of the macula.

Endocochlear potential. The large positive potential in the endolymph fluid created by its ionic composition. Changes in the endocochlear potential (usually a decrease) impair the transduction process and increase auditory thresholds.

Endolymph. One of the two fluids in the cochlear duct, the other one being perilymph. It has a unique ionic composition among extracellular body fluids (low Na^+, high K^+), which helps create the electrical gradient that drives the transduction process, the conversion of sound into nerve impulses.

Hair cells. The general term for the sensory cells in the cochlea and the vestibular system that carry out the transduction process, the conversion of sound into nerve impulses. Several types of hair cells can be morphologically and functionally distinguished. **Inner hair cells** are the primary transducers of sound in the cochlea; **outer hair cells** enhance transduction in the cochlea; **type I and type II hair cells** are part of the vestibular sensory apparatus.

Organ of Corti. The structure in the cochlea that houses the sensory cells (hair cells) and additional so-called supporting cells.

Spiral ganglion. The section of the cochlear nerve that directly innervates the hair cells.

Stria vascularis. A supporting structure in the cochlea. Its ion transport mechanisms create the ionic environment and electric potential of the endolymph.

REFERENCES

1. Schacht J, Hawkins JE. Sketches of otohistory. Part 11: Ototoxicity: drug-induced hearing loss. Audiol Neurootol 2006;11(1):1–6.

2. Scheifele P, Martin D, Clark JG, et al. Effect of kennel noise on hearing in dogs. Am J Vet Res 2012;73:482–9.
3. Schatz A, Bugie E, Waksman SA. Streptomycin, a substance exhibiting antibiotic activity against gram-positive and gram-negative bacteria. Proc Soc Exp Biol Med 1944;55:66–9.
4. Weinstein MJ, Luedemann GM, Oden EM, et al. Gentamicin, a new antibiotic complex from micromonospora. J Med Chem 1963;6:463–4.
5. Magnet S, Blanchard JS. Molecular insights into aminoglycoside action and resistance. Chem Rev 2005;105(2):477–98.
6. Lim SK, Nam HM, Kim A, et al. Detection and characterization of aparmycin-resistant Escherichia coli from humans in Korea. Microb Drug Resist 2011; 17(4):563–6.
7. Fischel-Ghodsian N. Genetic factors in aminoglycoside toxicity. Pharmacogenomics 2005;6(1):27–36.
8. Forge A, Schacht J. Aminoglycoside antibiotics. Audiol Neurootol 2000;5(1): 3–22.
9. Fee WE Jr. Aminoglycoside ototoxicity in the human. Laryngoscope 1980; 90(10 Pt 2 Suppl 24):1–19.
10. Lerner SA, Schmitt BA, Seligsohn R, et al. Comparative study of ototoxicity and nephrotoxicity in patients randomly assigned to treatment with amikacin or gentamicin. Am J Med 1986;80(6B):98–104.
11. Fausti SA, Henry JA, Schaffer HI, et al. High-frequency audiometric monitoring for early detection of aminoglycoside ototoxicity. J Infect Dis 1992;165(6): 1026–32.
12. de Jager P, van Altena R. Hearing loss and nephrotoxicity in long-term aminoglycoside treatment in patients with tuberculosis. Int J Tuberc Lung Dis 2002;6(7): 622–7.
13. Gookin JL, Riviere JE, Gilger BC, et al. Acute renal failure in four cats treated with paromomycin. J Am Vet Med Assoc 1999;215(12):1821–3, 1806.
14. European Agency for the Evaluation of Medicinal Products. Committee for veterinary medicinal products. Apramycin. Summary report (2). 1999. Available at: http://www.ema.europa.eu/docs/en_GB/document_library/Maximum_Residue_Limits_-_Report/2009/11/WC500010684.pdf. Accessed September 5, 2012.
15. Raphael Y, Fein A, Nebel L. Transplacental kanamycin ototoxicity in the guinea pig. Arch Otorhinolaryngol 1983;238(1):45–51.
16. Shepherd RK, Martin RL. Onset of ototoxicity in the cat is related to onset of auditory function. Hear Res 1995;92(1–2):131–42.
17. Henley CM, Rybak LP. Ototoxicity in developing mammals. Brain Res Brain Res Rev 1995;20(1):68–90.
18. Lenoir M, Marot M, Uziel A. Comparative ototoxicity of four aminoglycosidic antibiotics during the critical period of cochlear development in the rat. A functional and structural study. Acta Otolaryngol Suppl 1983;405:1–16.
19. Aran JM, Darrouzet J. Observation of click-evoked compound VIII nerve responses before, during, and over seven months after kanamycin treatment in the guinea pig. Acta Otolaryngol 1975;79(1–2):24–32.
20. Leake PA, Hradek GT. Cochlear pathology of long term neomycin induced deafness in cats. Hear Res 1988;33(1):11–33.
21. Pickrell JA, Oehme FW, Cash WC. Ototoxicity in dogs and cats. Semin Vet Med Surg (Small Anim) 1993;8(1):42–9.
22. Lindeman HH. Regional differences in sensitivity of the vestibular sensory epithelia to ototoxic antibiotics. Acta Otolaryngol 1969;67(2):177–89.

23. Wersall J, Hawkins JE Jr. The vestibular sensory epithelia in the cat labyrinth and their reactions in chronic streptomycin intoxication. Acta Otolaryngol 1962;54: 1–23.

24. Webster JC, McGee TM, Carroll R, et al. Ototoxicity of gentamicin. Histopathologic and functional results in the cat. Trans Am Acad Ophthalmol Otolaryngol 1970;74(6):1155–65.

25. Lautermann J, McLaren J, Schacht J. Glutathione protection against gentamicin ototoxicity depends on nutritional status. Hear Res 1995;86(1–2):15–24.

26. Clerici WJ, Hensley K, DiMartino DL, et al. Direct detection of ototoxicant-induced reactive oxygen species generation in cochlear explants. Hear Res 1996;98(1–2): 116–24.

27. Hirose K, Hockenbery DM, Rubel EW. Reactive oxygen species in chick hair cells after gentamicin exposure in vitro. Hear Res 1997;104(1–2):1–14.

28. Op de Beeck K, Schacht J, Van Camp G. Apoptosis in acquired and genetic hearing impairment: the programmed death of the hair cell. Hear Res 2011; 281(1–2):18–27.

29. Sha SH, Schacht J. Antioxidants attenuate gentamicin-induced free-radical formation in vitro and ototoxicity in vivo: D-methionine is a potential protectant. Hear Res 2000;142:34–40.

30. Sha SH, Qiu JH, Schacht J. Aspirin to prevent gentamicin-induced hearing loss. N Engl J Med 2006;354(17):1856–7.

31. Varzi HN, Esmailzadeh S, Morovvati H, et al. Effect of silymarin and vitamin E on gentamicin-induced nephrotoxicity in dogs. J Vet Pharmacol Ther 2007;30(5):477–81.

32. Rosenberg B. Platinum coordination complexes in cancer chemotherapy. Naturwissenschaften 1973;60(9):399–406.

33. Rozencweig M, von Hoff DD, Slavik M, et al. Cis-diamminedichloroplatinum (II). A new anticancer drug. Ann Intern Med 1977;86(6):803–12.

34. Benedetti Panici P, Greggi S, Scambia G, et al. Efficacy and toxicity of very high-dose cisplatin in advanced ovarian carcinoma: 4-year survival analysis and neurological follow-up. Int J Gynecol Cancer 1993;3(1):44–53.

35. Minami SB, Sha SH, Schacht J. Antioxidant protection in a new animal model of cisplatin-induced ototoxicity. Hear Res 2004;198(1–2):137–43.

36. Ravi R, Somani SM, Rybak LP. Mechanism of cisplatin ototoxicity: antioxidant system. Pharmacol Toxicol 1995;76(6):386–94.

37. Sergi B, Ferraresi A, Troiani D, et al. Cisplatin ototoxicity in the guinea pig: vestibular and cochlear damage. Hear Res 2003;182(1–2):56–64.

38. Stengs CH, Klis SF, Huizing EH, et al. Cisplatin ototoxicity. An electrophysiological dose-effect study in albino guinea pigs. Hear Res 1998;124(1–2):99–107.

39. van Ruijven MW, de Groot JC, Klis SF, et al. The cochlear targets of cisplatin: an electrophysiological and morphological time-sequence study. Hear Res 2005; 205(1–2):241–8.

40. Rybak LP, Whitworth CA, Mukherjea D, et al. Mechanisms of cisplatin-induced ototoxicity and prevention. Hear Res 2007;226(1–2):157–67.

41. Banfi B, Malgrange B, Knisz J, et al. NOX3, a superoxide-generating NADPH oxidase of the inner ear. J Biol Chem 2004;279(44):46065–72.

42. Alam SA, Ikeda K, Oshima T, et al. Cisplatin-induced apoptotic cell death in Mongolian gerbil cochlea. Hear Res 2000;141(1–2):28–38.

43. Mukherjea D, Jajoo S, Kaur T, et al. Transtympanic administration of short interfering (si)RNA for the NOX3 isoform of NADPH oxidase protects against cisplatin-induced hearing loss in the rat. Antioxid Redox Signal 2010;13(5): 589–98.

44. Mukherjea D, Jajoo S, Whitworth C, et al. Short interfering RNA against transient receptor potential vanilloid 1 attenuates cisplatin-induced hearing loss in the rat. J Neurosci 2008;28(49):13056–65.

45. Wang J, Ladrech S, Pujol R, et al. Caspase inhibitors, but not c-Jun NH2-terminal kinase inhibitor treatment, prevent cisplatin-induced hearing loss. Cancer Res 2004;64(24):9217–24.

46. Kang KP, Kim DH, Jung YJ, et al. Alpha-lipoic acid attenuates cisplatin-induced acute kidney injury in mice by suppressing renal inflammation. Nephrol Dial Transplant 2009;24(10):3012–20.

47. Choe WT, Chinosornvatana N, Chang KW. Prevention of cisplatin ototoxicity using transtympanic N-acetylcysteine and lactate. Otol Neurotol 2004;25(6):910–5.

48. Paksoy M, Ayduran E, Sanli A, et al. The protective effects of intratympanic dexamethasone and vitamin E on cisplatin-induced ototoxicity are demonstrated in rats. Med Oncol 2011;28(2):615–21.

49. Yildirim M, Inancli HM, Samanci B, et al. Preventing cisplatin induced ototoxicity by N-acetylcysteine and salicylate. Kulak Burun Bogaz Ihtis Derg 2010;20(4): 173–83.

50. Zarkovic N, Zarkovic K, Kralj M, et al. Anticancer and antioxidative effects of micronized zeolite clinoptilolite. Anticancer Res 2003;23(2B):1589–95.

51. Winter JL, Barber LG, Freeman L, et al. Antioxidant status and biomarkers of oxidative stress in dogs with lymphoma. J Vet Intern Med 2009;23(2):311–6.

52. Williams JH. The use of gamma linolenic acid, linoleic acid and natural vitamin E for the treatment of multicentric lymphoma in two dogs. J S Afr Vet Assoc 1988; 59(3):141–4.

53. Greenlee H, Hershman DL, Jacobson JS. Use of antioxidant supplements during breast cancer treatment: a comprehensive review. Breast Cancer Res Treat 2009; 115(3):437–52.

54. Whitworth C, Morris C, Scott V, et al. Dose-response relationships for furosemide ototoxicity in rat. Hear Res 1993;71(1–2):202–7.

55. Rybak LP, Whitworth C, Scott V. Comparative acute ototoxicity of loop diuretic compounds. Eur Arch Otorhinolaryngol 1991;248(6):353–7.

56. Li Y, Ding D, Jiang H, et al. Co-administration of cisplatin and furosemide causes rapid and massive loss of cochlear hair cells in mice. Neurotox Res 2011;20(4): 307–19.

57. Rybak LP. Pathophysiology of furosemide ototoxicity. J Otolaryngol 1982;11(2): 127–33.

58. Brummett RE. Ototoxicity resulting from the combined administration of potent diuretics and other agents. Scand Audiol Suppl 1981;14(Suppl):215–24.

59. Hirose K, Sato E. Comparative analysis of combination kanamycin-furosemide versus kanamycin alone in the mouse cochlea. Hear Res 2011;272(1–2):108–16.

60. Rybak LP. Furosemide ototoxicity: clinical and experimental aspects. Laryngoscope 1985;95(9 Pt 2 Suppl 38):1–14.

61. Brown RD. Comparative acute cochlear toxicity of intravenous bumetanide and furosemide in the purebred beagle. J Clin Pharmacol 1981;21(11–12 Pt 2): 620–7.

62. Sewell WF. The relation between the endocochlear potential and spontaneous activity in auditory nerve fibres of the cat. J Physiol 1984;347:685–96.

63. Gottl KH, Roesch A, Klinke R. Quantitative evaluation of ototoxic side effects of furosemide, piretanide, bumetanide, azosemide and ozolinone in the cat–a new approach to the problem of ototoxicity. Naunyn Schmiedebergs Arch Pharmacol 1985;331(2–3):275–82.

64. Brown RD, Manno JE, Daigneault EA, et al. Comparative acute ototoxicity of intravenous bumetanide and furosemide in the pure-bred beagle. Toxicol Appl Pharmacol 1979;48(1 Pt 1):157–69.
65. Mathog RH, Thomas WG, Hudson WR. Ototoxicity of new and potent diuretics. A preliminary study. Arch Otolaryngol 1970;92(1):7–13.
66. Goldman WJ, Bielinski TC, Mattis PA. Cochlear microphonic potential response of the dog to diuretic compounds. Toxicol Appl Pharmacol 1973;25(2):259–66.
67. Forge A. Observations on the stria vascularis of the guinea pig cochlea and the changes resulting from the administration of the diuretic furosemide. Clin Otolaryngol Allied Sci 1976;1(3):211–9.
68. Arnold W, Nadol JB Jr, Weidauer H. Ultrastructural histopathology in a case of human ototoxicity due to loop diuretics. Acta Otolaryngol 1981;91(5–6):399–414.
69. Rybak LP, Whitworth C, Scott V, et al. Ototoxicity of furosemide during development. Laryngoscope 1991;101(11):1167–74.
70. Brusilow SW. Propranolol antagonism to the effect of furosemide on the composition of endolymph in guinea pigs. Can J Physiol Pharmacol 1976;54(1):42–8.
71. Rybak LP, Whitworth C. Some organic acids attenuate the effects of furosemide on the endocochlear potential. Hear Res 1987;26(1):89–93.

Index

Vet Clin Small Anim 42 (2012) 1273–1283
http://dx.doi.org/10.1016/S0195-5616(12)00177-5
0195-5616/12/$ – see front matter © 2012 Elsevier Inc. All rights reserved.

vetsmall.theclinics.com

United States Postal Service
Statement of Ownership, Management, and Circulation
(All Periodicals Publications Except Requestor Publications)

1. Publication Title	2. Publication Number	3. Filing Date
Veterinary Clinics of North America: Small Animal Practice	0 0 3 - 1 5 0	9/14/12

4. Issue Frequency	5. Number of Issues Published Annually	6. Annual Subscription Price
Jan, Mar, May, Jul, Sep, Nov	6	$283.00

7. Complete Mailing Address of Known Office of Publication (Not printer) (Street, city, county, state, and ZIP+4®)

Elsevier Inc.
360 Park Avenue South
New York, NY 10010-1710

Contact Person
Stephen Bushing

Telephone (Include area code)
215-239-3688

8. Complete Mailing Address of Headquarters or General Business Office of Publisher (Not printer)

Elsevier Inc., 360 Park Avenue South, New York, NY 10010-1710

9. Full Names and Complete Mailing Addresses of Publisher, Editor, and Managing Editor (Do not leave blank)
Publisher (Name and complete mailing address)

Kim Murphy, Elsevier, Inc., 1600 John F. Kennedy Blvd. Suite 1800, Philadelphia, PA 19103-2899

Editor (Name and complete mailing address)

John Vassallo, Elsevier, Inc., 1600 John F. Kennedy Blvd. Suite 1800, Philadelphia, PA 19103-2899

Managing Editor (Name and complete mailing address)

Barbara Cohen-Kligerman, Elsevier, Inc., 1600 John F. Kennedy Blvd. Suite 1800, Philadelphia, PA 19103-2899

10. Owner (Do not leave blank. If the publication is owned by a corporation, give the name and address of the corporation immediately followed by the names and addresses of all stockholders owning or holding 1 percent or more of the total amount of stock. If not owned by a corporation, give the names and addresses of the individual owners. If owned by a partnership or other unincorporated firm, give its name and address as well as those of each individual owner. If the publication is published by a nonprofit organization, give its name and address.)

Full Name	Complete Mailing Address
Wholly owned subsidiary of	1600 John F. Kennedy Blvd., Ste. 1800
Reed/Elsevier, US holdings	Philadelphia, PA 19103-2899

11. Known Bondholders, Mortgagees, and Other Security Holders Owning or Holding 1 Percent or More of Total Amount of Bonds, Mortgages, or Other Securities. If none, check box ☐ None

Full Name	Complete Mailing Address
N/A	

12. Tax Status (For completion by nonprofit organizations authorized to mail at nonprofit rates) (Check one)
The purpose, function, and nonprofit status of this organization and the exempt status for federal income tax purposes:
☐ Has Not Changed During Preceding 12 Months
☐ Has Changed During Preceding 12 Months (Publisher must submit explanation of change with this statement)

PS Form 3526, September 2007 (Page 1 of 3 (Instructions Page 3)) PSN 7530-01-000-9931 PRIVACY NOTICE: See our Privacy policy in www.usps.com

13. Publication Title	14. Issue Date for Circulation Data Below
Veterinary Clinics of North America: Small Animal Practice	July 2012

15. Extent and Nature of Circulation		Average No. Copies Each Issue During Preceding 12 Months	No. Copies of Single Issue Published Nearest to Filing Date
a. Total Number of Copies (Net press run)		1757	1546
b. Paid Circulation (By Mail and Outside the Mail)	(1) Mailed Outside-County Paid Subscriptions Stated on PS Form 3541. (Include paid distribution above nominal rate, advertiser's proof copies, and exchange copies)	1092	1007
	(2) Mailed In-County Paid Subscriptions Stated on PS Form 3541 (Include paid distribution above nominal rate, advertiser's proof copies, and exchange copies)		
	(3) Paid Distribution Outside the Mails Including Sales Through Dealers and Carriers, Street Vendors, Counter Sales, and Other Paid Distribution Outside USPS®	270	253
	(4) Paid Distribution by Other Classes Mailed Through the USPS (e.g. First-Class Mail®)		
c. Total Paid Distribution (Sum of 15b (1), (2), (3), and (4)) ▲		1362	1260
d. Free or Nominal Rate Distribution (By Mail and Outside the Mail)	(1) Free or Nominal Rate Outside-County Copies Included on PS Form 3541	97	105
	(2) Free or Nominal Rate In-County Copies Included on PS Form 3541		
	(3) Free or Nominal Rate Copies Mailed at Other Classes Through the USPS (e.g. First-Class Mail)		
	(4) Free or Nominal Rate Distribution Outside the Mail (Carriers or other means)		
e. Total Free or Nominal Rate Distribution (Sum of 15d (1), (2), (3) and (4)) ▲		97	105
f. Total Distribution (Sum of 15c and 15e) ▲		1459	1365
g. Copies not Distributed (See instructions to publishers #4 (page #3)) ▲		298	181
h. Total (Sum of 15f and g) ▲		1757	1546
i. Percent Paid (15c divided by 15f times 100)		93.35%	92.31%

16. Publication of Statement of Ownership
If the publication is a general publication, publication of this statement is required. Will be printed in the November 2012 issue of this publication.

☐ Publication not required

17. Signature and Title of Editor, Publisher, Business Manager, or Owner

Stephen R. Bushing

Stephen R. Bushing –Inventory Distribution Coordinator

Date: September 14, 2012

I certify that all information furnished on this form is true and complete. I understand that anyone who furnishes false or misleading information on this form or who omits material or information requested on the form may be subject to criminal sanctions (including fines and imprisonment) and/or civil sanctions (including civil penalties).

Moving?

Make sure your subscription moves with you!

To notify us of your new address, find your **Clinics Account Number** (located on your mailing label above your name), and contact customer service at:

Email: journalscustomerservice-usa@elsevier.com

800-654-2452 (subscribers in the U.S. & Canada)
314-447-8871 (subscribers outside of the U.S. & Canada)

Fax number: 314-447-8029

Elsevier Health Sciences Division
Subscription Customer Service
3251 Riverport Lane
Maryland Heights, MO 63043

*To ensure uninterrupted delivery of your subscription, please notify us at least 4 weeks in advance of move.

Printed and bound by CPI Group (UK) Ltd, Croydon, CR0 4YY

03/10/2024

01040442-0015